Reboot with Joe
FULLY CHARGED

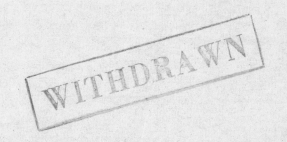

Reboot with Joe
FULLY CHARGED
Seven keys to losing weight, staying healthy & thriving

Joe Cross

HODDER

First published in Great Britain in 2015 by Hodder & Stoughton

An Hachette UK company

This edition first published in 2016

1

A CIP catalogue record for this title
is available from the British Library

Paperback ISBN 9781473613485
Ebook ISBN 9781473613478

Typeset in Scala and Rockwell by Palimpsest Book Production Limited,
Falkirk, Stirlingshire

Printed and bound by CPI Group (UK) Ltd, Croydon CR0 4YY

Hodder & Stoughton policy is to use papers that are natural, renewable
and recyclable products and made from wood grown in sustainable forests.
The logging and manufacturing processes are expected to conform to the
environmental regulations of the country of origin.

Hodder & Stoughton Ltd
Carmelite House
50 Victoria Embankment
London EC4Y 0DZ

www.hodder.co.uk

This book is dedicated to the Reboot community – those of you with a love of plants, who share your successes and setbacks, sage advice and unflagging encouragement and support with so many, including me.

Contents

Acknowledgements

Thank you to:

The 20 million-plus viewers of *Fat, Sick & Nearly Dead*, who've seen the film and spread the word.

The one million-plus and counting members of the Reboot community, who continue to inspire and motivate so many, including me. You've created a movement.

The Reboot team – Jamin Mendelsohn, Kari Thorstensen, Susan Ainsworth, Amie Hannon, Shane Hodson, Brenna Ryan, Jamie Schneider, Sophie Carrel, Chris Zilo, Ameet Maturu, Alex Tibbetts, Erin Flowers, Sarah Mawson, Lisa Merkle, Grace Ha, Sean Frechette, Kristen DeAngelis, Vernon Caldwell and Kurt Engfehr – who put their hearts and souls into nurturing the Reboot community and supporting the mission of Reboot with Joe.

My experts – Dr Shelia Kar, Dr Dean Ornish, Dr Brian Wansink and Dr Russell Kennedy – who generously gave of their time and shared their knowledge on how to sustain weight loss and stay healthy.

Barry Jacinto, Bobby Brennan, Carrie Diulus MD, Christopher Treloar, Ciruu Kiniti, Kate Elinsky, Michael Kyles-Villalobos and Phil Staples for your willingness to share your stories.

Our Reboot nutritionists – Stacy Kennedy, Claire Georgiou, Isabel Smith, Abigail Hueber, Rachel Gargano and Rhaya

Jordan – who have patiently coached Rebooters, answered questions and given advice on www.rebootwithjoe.com.

The Reboot with Joe Medical Advisory Board – in addition to Stacy Kennedy and Carrie Diulus MD, Ronald Penny MD, DSc and Adrian J. Rawlinson MD – for keeping the facts straight and for advocating the benefits of Rebooting.

J.P. Faber for helping to write this book – translating hours of conversation into a manuscript and providing research and insight.

Sarah Hammond and the team at Hodder & Stoughton and the team at Greenleaf Book Group for their guidance and enthusiasm in bringing this book to market.

Juice on!

Foreword

Mark Hyman MD

We in America have a problem with our weight and we are not alone. Almost 70 per cent of Americans are overweight, along with a third of the entire planet – about 2.1 billion people – triple the number in 1980. This is causing havoc with our collective health, and is responsible for a litany of 'lifestyle' illnesses that are the leading causes of death: coronary disease, cancer, stroke, diabetes – even dementia. According to the World Health Organization, excess fat is now behind 80 per cent of world health-care costs and comes with a global price tag of $47 trillion over the next 20 years.

In light of this stunning and continuing expansion of our waistlines, the question that begs to be asked is 'Why?' Why do so many of us eat food we know isn't good for us, causing us to gain weight and aggravate the symptoms of chronic illnesses? What exactly is so broken that we can't fix ourselves, choosing instead to consume substances known to destroy our lives?

In my own studies on the subject, which I have written about in *The Blood Sugar Solution* and *The Blood Sugar Solution 10-Day Detox Diet*, I've come to the conclusion that food addiction has a huge part to play. Preying upon our genetically wired attraction to anything sweet, the industrial food-makers have engineered food products that are literally more addictive than cocaine. We just can't seem to stop eating food that's laden with sugar, and we consume enormous amounts of it – an average of 22 teaspoons a day per person in the USA, with the rest of the West in fast pursuit (the average Briton eats 20 teaspoons a day, while the average Australian manages 18). Artificial sweeteners are just as bad for us, triggering the same health problems.

So what's to be done? The first thing we need to do is break the cycle of food addiction. Until you fix that, with a diet of whole, real, fresh food, anything else you do isn't going to matter much. And while that sounds simple enough, it's a tough task because addictive sugars and sweeteners are everywhere, in everything from spaghetti sauce to flavoured yogurt. What makes me furious as a doctor is to see patients who blame themselves for food addiction, and who believe it's their own lack of will-power that's at fault. The truth of the matter is that your brain, along with your hormones and taste buds, has been hijacked by the trillion-dollar processed food industry.

One of the things I've always liked about Joe Cross is his fundamental insight that we can break our addiction to scientifically engineered 'Frankenfoods' with a Reboot diet of whole plant-foods and juice. This will reset our brains and our biology back to a natural state.

But that is just half the battle. Anyone familiar with the diet industry knows that most people return to their old ways, and once again fall prey to the tricks and traps set by the food industry, everything from addictive chemicals to environmental inducements, such as advertising and pretty packaging.

In this book Joe confronts the challenge of what it takes to maintain a healthy lifestyle after the Reboot, based as usual on his own personal experience. What I admire is his profound understanding that you need a sustainable strategy for good health and weight loss that balances your brain chemistry without putting you into starvation mode or a dietary straitjacket. What he gets is that it's not about a short-term fix, but about changing your long-term habits and ways of thinking about food.

The changes and suggestions that Joe offers here are designed to create a deeper understanding of why we eat the way we do, and what it takes to change these habits permanently and build a new lifestyle that embraces a healthy diet. Incorporating these ideas will go a long way towards permanently freeing us all from food addiction and giving us back control over our own health. Read on.

Introduction

'Do you eat?'

There it is, the question I get asked at every event. 'Look at me,' I reply, 'of course I eat.' This is followed by 'What do you eat?' And, truth be told, I'm a little uncomfortable with that question, though I'm asked it all the time.

I'm quite comfortable telling my Reboot story. Anyone who has seen *Fat, Sick & Nearly Dead* knows that. It's my story of losing 7 stone (100 pounds) and a painful auto-immune disease by rejecting my bad lifestyle choices and running back into the embrace of Mother Nature, juicing and eating only plants.

The film became a hit, now seen by an estimated 20 million people. Since its launch, I've pretty much spent my time travelling and spreading the word about juicing and the power of fruits and veggies. So, then, why does it make me uncomfortable when people ask 'What do you eat now?'

Maybe because I'm not perfect. I struggle. I'm not the expert. I'm like most of you. Stress gets to me, I reach for my comfort foods, I don't exercise like I should, I have trouble sleeping, my weight fluctuates. I'm the poster guy for eating your veggies and it's still hard for me. But that's my challenge – to figure out how to keep on being healthy.

I call the distance from your hand to your mouth 'the last two feet of freedom'. You are the one controlling what you put in your mouth. It's free choice. But why we make the choices we do is complicated. It's not that we don't know that fruits and veggies are good for us. We all know that. But most of the time we don't eat them like we should.

I get to meet a great many success stories when I'm on the road. They are incredibly inspiring. And what I always ask these people – what I zero in on – is the question of how they sustain healthy habits. If it's hard for me (and I work on this all the time), it must be really hard for them. What gives them the strength to continue, and not fall back into old ways? What lets them sustain and even thrive?

What I've learned is that what works for me is not necessarily what works for everybody. I know what I should eat, but every individual has their own diet that is best for them. With this exception: that everyone needs a lot of plants in their diet to stay healthy. Also, that staying healthy and keeping the weight off is not just about what you eat. It's about *why* you eat what you eat. It's about all the psychological reasons why we struggle and why we self-destruct.

I don't have all the answers for how I should stay healthy. I'm finding out as I go along, and I think I'm getting better at it. I also don't have all the answers for how everyone else should stay healthy. But I've learned a great deal, and that's what I intend to share with you in this book.

Fat, Sick & Nearly Dead was a film about my journey to health. The sequel, *Fat, Sick & Nearly Dead 2,* and this book is about how we might stay 'there' in that happy place when we arrive at the end of the journey. Or maybe the journey doesn't really end, and it's my search for the answer to the question of how we can continue with a healthy, happy life.

So back to that question. What do I eat? I try to eat mostly plants. This is what I call a PLANT-BASED diet. I am not plant-only, I am plant-based. Every day is different; if it weren't, I'd get bored. I like my juice and I like my smoothies. I really do love salad and I'm not just saying that. Veggies are great but I'm not big on all of them. As an example, I'd much prefer to juice a cucumber than eat it. I eat animal protein, mostly something from the sea or chicken. I stay light on the red meat. I don't drink alcohol. I very rarely have a soda, and if I do, it's a ginger ale on a special occasion. I don't drink coffee or tea. But I love a good vegan soup. Of course, with my sweet tooth I love almost everything containing chocolate, be it cookies, cakes, ice cream or milkshakes. I try my best to have these in moderation. Most of the time I succeed, but there are definitely times when I don't. I'm not perfect. But then I don't know anyone who is.

Part I
THE PUZZLE OF REAL FOOD, REAL LIFE

THE JOURNEY CONTINUES

My name is Joe Cross. I am not a doctor, a nutritionist, a scientist, or even a journalist. I am just a guy who eight years ago reached a point where he couldn't stand it any longer. Thanks to a lifestyle rich in junk food and calories, along with booze, cigarettes and zero exercise, my stomach was so large it looked like I'd swallowed a sheep. My condition was made all the worse by a painful autoimmune disease called urticaria, which caused me to break out in hives from the slightest touch, and required taking nasty prescription drugs on a daily basis.

If you've seen my film *Fat, Sick & Nearly Dead*, you know I was able to change my life. I lost nearly 7 stone (100 pounds) and cured my illness by drinking nothing but fresh-pressed fruit and vegetable juice for 60 days, followed by three months of a plant-only diet. I called the time period of consuming only fruits and vegetables a Reboot because, rather like rebooting a computer, my whole system was reset, from my metabolism to my taste buds.

Eight years ago the idea of going on a juice-only diet for 60 days was pretty drastic. It still is, but eight years ago the world had not discovered juicing – juice bars were scarce, and you couldn't order an online 'cleanse' to be delivered to your door. Most people thought I was bonkers. But hitting 23 stone (320 pounds) and suffering from a miserable, debilitating disease left me willing to try something drastic.

Most doctors today agree that about 70 per cent of all disease is caused by lifestyle choices.[1] The big three are what you choose to eat and drink, how much you choose to exercise, and whether or not you choose to smoke. I was the poster boy for bad choices. I ate and drank with abandon – fast food, fried foods, sodas, pizza, burgers, fries, ice cream, beer and spirits. I smoked. And exercise? Well, I liked to think I was the same athletic rugby player of my youth, but, in truth, for years the closest I got to a rugby pitch was the distance from my TV to the couch.

So I thought, if I was lucky and within that 70 per cent, my illness would prove to be caused by my lifestyle choices. I knew I had turned my back on Mother Nature. I had only the most glancing relationship with green vegetables – those were the things I moved to the side to get to what I actually wanted – and 'fruit' was most often the maraschino cherry atop a sundae or a handful of berries decorating a plate of *real* dessert. What would happen if I embraced Mother Nature? What if I took my fruit and vegetable intake from zero to 100 per cent? I decided to find out.

If you've seen *Fat, Sick & Nearly Dead*, you know that by the end of my journey I was medication-free. I had lost more than 7 stone (100 pounds) and was full of energy and vitality. I felt like I was on top of the world. What I didn't know was that the Reboot I had just completed was the easy part!

The first hurdle

My transformation in *Fat, Sick & Nearly Dead* was supposed to be the whole story. I had decided to film my Reboot, thinking that filming would make me stick to it. My plan and hope was that my Reboot journey would end with me in a new state of health. (If it didn't, at least I'd have the satisfaction of knowing I'd given it my best shot.) I'd return to Australia, pick up my life as a businessman, release a film that only my friends and family would see, and live happily and healthily ever after.

Things were going according to plan. The Reboot worked. I was back in Australia weighing 15½ stone (220 pounds), and I was medication-free, eating plants and exercising. I resumed my business of investing and entrepreneurship, and I was finishing the film. I was healthy and happy. Then I received a phone call that changed everything.

Six months after I completed my Reboot and was back in Australia, I got a call from a truck driver named Phil Staples. I had met him at a truck stop in Arizona while filming *Fat, Sick & Nearly Dead*. At over 28 stone (400 pounds) and suffering from the same auto-immune disorder as me, I felt an immediate affinity with Phil. We talked and shared Phil's first-ever green juice. I told him to call me if he ever needed help.

To my surprise, Phil accepted my offer. 'You gave me your card about six months ago and I need help,' he told me on the phone. 'Will you help me? You promised you would.' I had made that promise to Phil and I knew I had to help him. I suggested a Reboot, which Phil agreed to; he also agreed to be filmed.

Honestly, I didn't think that Phil would do it, but I thought we could at least film him and put him in the credits of our movie. I really thought he wouldn't go for more than four or five days of juicing – if he would even be allowed to do that much by his doctors. Boy, was I wrong.

In a process that took the better part of a year, Phil completely changed his life. At the end of the year he had lost almost 14 stone (200 pounds) and was healthier and better looking than he had been in years. Like me, he'd also cured his auto-immune disease. What's more, he was active in his local community and in many ways living a healthy, happy life.

What I couldn't foresee at the time was that Phil's decision to follow me on a Reboot journey and change his life would have a profound impact on my own. Instead of fading into the sunset as a healthy, happy and successful Australian businessman, I would have a hit film, travel non-stop spreading the word of juicing for health, and found my own wellness company. My own weight would fluctuate from 15½ stone (220 pounds) to a high of 18½ stone (260 pounds) and I would struggle to maintain my new-found health.

The addition of Phil to the film turned out to be a great thing from the point of view of the film itself. It showed that I was not unique in my struggle to be healthy or in my ability to achieve a new, healthy lifestyle and rid myself of a debilitating disease. It also made me realize that I had something important to share with a lot of people – that it is truly possible to harness the power of plants to transform ourselves into happier and healthier people. It made me see that I'd really hit on something a lot more important than my own personal struggle.

I also realized that Phil gave the film its heart and soul. Here's a truck driver from Iowa, an ordinary guy everybody could identify with. As an Aussie businessman, there's nothing about me nearly as inspiring as Phil. He's the one with the message – that anybody, no matter how desperate they have become, can turn things around with a Reboot.

With the addition of Phil, it seemed like I now had a film that could be more than a 'friends and family' screening. I started working on how it could be released to as large an audience as possible. It was something I had never done before, in an industry I had no experience with, but, as with the Reboot, I was ready to give it my best shot. But it also became my first hurdle in maintaining a healthy, happy Joe.

You see, before I got that phone call from Phil, my film was basically done. It was on budget, on time, on schedule, and everything was hunky dory. Starting the journey with Phil meant shooting and editing basically a whole new film. And because that was 2008, the timing couldn't have been worse. The whole world was cascading into recession and economic crisis, and the Australian dollar in particular crashed against the US dollar. So not only did the budget double on paper, it quadrupled for me because of the currency effect.

Even with the stress of a growing film budget, I managed to keep my weight in check. After we wrapped up the filming of Phil's transformation in mid-2009, I spent the rest of that year either at home in Sydney or in New York, where I worked in an editing room in the West Village or in our small, three-person staff office in Brooklyn. I laboured hard but there was routine. I got up in the morning, worked out, walked past my favourite juice bar on the way to work, had my list of restaurants with good whole-plant meals, and slept in the same bed every night.

And these healthy habits showed in my waistline. Although

I put on 10 pounds during the year we filmed Phil – not unexpectedly because most people regain some weight after any diet – during the editing of the film I lost them again and was back to my bantam weight.

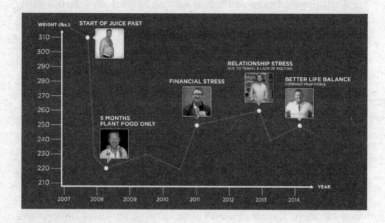

Growing pains

The first cracks in my armour of health and happiness started to appear in 2010. Money had become a serious problem. In addition to the extended filming time for Phil, further delays pushed the launch date from late 2010 to early 2011. I had to pay for post-production and, of course, pay everyone. At the same time, other investments I'd made in my previous life as a businessman were in crisis and needed attention and more funding. I had too many holes to plug in the financial dam, with cash leaking out daily. No revenue was coming in from the film, which nobody even knew about. It was still just 95 or 96 minutes of digital images on a video drive somewhere in the ether.

To say that life had become stressful is like saying it's a

little humid outside in the middle of a monsoon. Back while I was actually on my journey of juicing, and especially after I'd completed my first Reboot, I was in great shape, in a great headspace. I found that I didn't really have to think too much about being healthy. I had a new love of fruits and vegetables, and my body actually craved those fruits and vegetables. I no longer wanted to eat pizza and burgers. I had quit smoking and drinking, and I had a regular exercise regime. My life was balanced and I had a routine. I also thought I had kicked my addiction to sugar and fat.

Now I was like a prizefighter getting pummelled into the corner. And what was my response? How did I cope? I ran to my old friend, *sugar!* I went right back to the comfort foods of my childhood, when I would get home after school, eat sugar cereal and watch TV. To this day, when I am stressed out or unhappy or lonely I crave sugar. So although I've never stopped my daily juices since my journey began, I went to sugar a few too many times. By the time the film was ready for showing, my weight had increased to 17½ stone (245 pounds).

Still, the film was done and it got a great reception. I started a grassroots campaign, showing it at festivals and in small venues to small audiences who were already interested in health and wellness. The feedback left me full of energy and encouragement, and my grassroots effort paid off: the film was picked up by Netflix, which launched it to their audience in July 2011.

I was not expecting the explosion that came next. To my surprise, *Fat, Sick & Nearly Dead* became an overnight sensation. Literally millions of people watched it. For the first two or three months after the launch you couldn't get a juicer anywhere in the USA: retailers large and small simply couldn't meet demand. Even the *Wall Street Journal* picked up on the sensation, with an article about my effect on juicer sales and the impact that *Fat, Sick & Nearly Dead* had had in the retail sector.

So, with a hit on my hands, I went back on the road, figuring I had to take advantage of the movie going viral. And I loved it. Like my grassroots campaign, I enjoyed the touching and talking to people and the storytelling. It was great fun. But it was more than that; people were really giving me a lot of buoyancy with their enthusiasm. Lots of energy was coming my way, and I was starting to learn how to take that energy from the community and utilize it to my advantage – to have it become my support and my inspiration. This came as a revelation: that getting up in front of a crowd and talking about my experience helped reinforce what I should be doing. As I discovered, there was no better way to learn than to teach and share.

But it wasn't all roses. The amazing success of the film unleashed its own tsunami of stress. All those people who'd seen the film and gone out and bought juicers? They wanted more information. They wanted help. They wanted to succeed. They wanted to know what to do and when to do it and how to do it. They wanted to know how they should store juice, how much juice they should drink each day, what they should do if they felt light-headed, why they were losing weight, what to do about protein, and so on.

Before the Netflix release, I spent a considerable amount investing in 'infrastructure', hiring Reboot nutritionist Stacy Kennedy to create Reboot plans and answer questions. I also built a community website that was supposed to provide people with all the support and information they needed to successfully Reboot. But it couldn't handle the traffic we generated, which grew exponentially. Our community increased to over 300,000 and the website crashed.

Talk about pressure and a feeling of failure! Here I was with a big, broken website and in a financial hole. This was not how I'd envisioned things playing out. But, like most things in life, very little turns out exactly as planned. What you have to do is adjust, regroup and come at it again – have another go at it, as we say Down Under.

I worked hard all of 2012, under tremendous financial pressure, but before the year was out I'd found investors who liked the film and the vision of what we wanted to accomplish, and who believed we could build a sustainable company. I was able to bring on a great team to help me put together the right online platform, and to help with all the expertise I needed in terms of nutrition and lifestyle advice. My only problem by the end of the year was my weight. I was still cured of my illness and free from the need to take any pills, but I had crept back up to 18½ stone (260 pounds).

Part of this came from the travelling. Now, I like to travel, and I love meeting people who've been inspired by my story – it's what inspires me. But travelling all the time brought a new level of strain. I was experiencing what so many people face – having to hold down jobs, raise families and take care of all their other commitments – the challenge of finding time for healthy habits. I couldn't seem to carve out time to go to the gym, to be relaxed, to take a walk in the park, or to go and look at how beautiful the world of nature was.

My personal relationships were also suffering. I couldn't sustain a long-distance relationship with my girlfriend in Australia, someone I cared for deeply. I had family pressure, with my mother and father saying, 'We never see you, Joe.'

I was disconnected from friends in Australia and New York; it was like, 'We don't invite you any more because you're never here. Why send you an invitation to our party when you won't come?' Hearing this kind of thing when I flew home made me feel like a stranger. It was like I'd dropped off the face of the Earth into some hole where I just worked all the time.

This was something I didn't fit into my formula. I know that being an entrepreneur is about taking risks, making sacrifices and being passionate about what you do. But the life of an entrepreneur can also be incredibly lonely.

What kept me going was something I also wasn't expecting: the support of the community all around me. That enthusiasm and realizing I'd found my passion are what sustained me. I knew that many, many people out there were in the same position as me – under stress, hurting and trying to keep it together. I thought it was worth having somebody out there who wasn't an 'expert', but rather one of them, championing the way with an 'If I can do it, you can do it' attitude. I didn't want to let them down.

It was also a little bit scary to go back to 18½ stone (260 pounds). Here I was with a movie about my success at losing a mountain of weight and, my God, look what was happening to me! Sure, I'd been facing a perfect storm of stress from too little money, too much travel, and too much loneliness, but this was double trouble – being a poster boy for wellness who couldn't stop eating sugar!

Despite the sugar, I was still eating what I consider a healthy diet – juice, smoothies, and salads, lots of fruits, vegetables and wholegrains. And I was still healthy – medication-free, no signs of my urticaria. But I didn't look so healthy. The problem was that I had been looking at my health one-dimensionally. I was singularly focused on my diet – what I was eating. What I learned is that if you don't make time to exercise, to sleep and to enjoy life – if you don't have balance in your life – it's hard to maintain your health.

I'd slipped into some pretty unhealthy habits and needed to correct course. One thing I say about a Reboot is that it's always there if you need to reset your system. So I started 2013 with a 15-day Reboot, and over the course of the next few months focused on achieving a better balance – dealing with stress, making time to exercise and getting enough rest. I got my weight back down to 17 stone (240 pounds), which is where I have been, more or less, ever since.

And to tell you the truth, I'm pretty happy with my weight right there. I'm also pretty happy with life. Despite the stresses of the last seven years, it's been an amazing journey to places I never imagined when I was travelling across the US, drinking my juice. I was able to take my new-found passion for health and wellness and make it my life. And, above everything else, I have my health.

Do I still struggle? Absolutely. I went on the road for my last book tour, and four months took their toll. I tried to fit in every request for an appearance from Liverpool, to Vancouver, to Orlando, to Kansas City, to Seattle, to Santa Cruz. It was hard carving out time for myself, and after four months I was tired. But I've learned to recognize when my life is getting out of balance, and what it takes to bring it back. Through my travels, through my struggles, through my meetings with wellness experts, through listening to the stories of so many successful Rebooters, I've learned the steps that I need to stay where I want to be – healthy and happy.

When I completed *Fat, Sick & Nearly Dead*, I had no intention of making another film, but I realized that there was much more to know. The journey didn't stop at the end of the Reboot. Sustaining health and wellness is a lifelong challenge. *Fat, Sick & Nearly Dead 2* and this book are the continuation of my story and the continuation of the stories of the thousands of Rebooters I've met. I thought it was essential to share what I'd learned because if I can do it, and if I can slip and fall, and get back up and on track, if I can sustain my success . . . guess what? You can too.

LESSONS LEARNED

It's been eight years now since I began my journey with juicing and my love affair with plants. As you can imagine, I've learned an enormous amount since then, not only about myself and about nutrition, but also about staying healthy in an unhealthy world.

When we made the first *Fat, Sick & Nearly Dead* film, I'll admit that I was an amateur. I knew nothing about nutrition. I didn't even know if juicing would cure my illness and get me off medication. It did (thank you, Mother Nature), but if you saw the movie, you were watching someone who didn't know what he was doing.

I also knew nothing about making a film. I didn't know how to edit, release, distribute or publicize it. I especially didn't know the film would inspire hundreds of thousands of people to Reboot, so I didn't know I'd face an avalanche of questions, such as: What about protein? What do I do if I'm feeling nauseous? Is it OK to drink juice if I have Hashimoto's disease? What if I have diabetes – can I Reboot? If my doctor doesn't support this, can I Reboot? It went on from there.

So I did what I always do when I don't know the answers. I went to the experts and the community around me. I worked with seasoned film veterans, I found a distribution company willing to take on the film, and I brought on board

Stacy Kennedy and Claire Georgiou as the Reboot nutritionists to develop plans and answer questions. On our website we started publishing success stories to inspire others and share 'how I did it' advice. And I asked lots and lots of questions.

But the biggest thing I didn't know when I finished my Reboot and was sitting on top of the world was this: *losing weight and getting healthy was the easy part. Keeping it off and staying healthy is the hard part.*

I guess if I had thought about it, I would have known this. As Reboot nutritionist Stacy Kennedy likes to point out, there is no shortage of people losing weight. At any given time, something like 43 million Americans alone are on a diet. The reality is that most of these people – anywhere from 65 to 98 per cent, depending on the research source – will regain the weight they lose within 12 months. The weight-loss industry makes $60 billion a year. You don't get to that 'size' if people are successful at sustaining their weight loss.

Had I thought about it before I started my Reboot, I would have known that the odds of succeeding and healing myself were slim. If I'd thought about it even more, I'd have known that the odds of sustaining that success were even slimmer. But I was fresh to all of this, and full of the confidence that comes with starting something new. If I'd thought about it enough, I probably wouldn't have even begun. But I did, and it worked – at least at first.

So here I was, travelling non-stop as the poster boy for Rebooting, struggling with sustaining my own weight loss and health, and talking to thousands of people who were just getting started on a Reboot, or who had just successfully completed one and were sitting on top of the mountain. I knew that soon they'd have the same questions I did. What do I do now? Now that I've got fit, how can I sustain it?

So what did I do? Again, I turned to the experts and my community in search of answers. And I made a second movie about it: *Fat, Sick & Nearly Dead 2*. I learned loads of useful information, which this book shares with you. Above all, I learned that the answer is not a simple one.

KIVDI (Knowing it versus doing it)

I try to live my life according to a few basic principles, the first of which is that honesty will set you free. This sounds like the lyrics to some folk song, but what I mean is that it's always better to be honest with yourself and with others. It saves a lot of time and heartache.

I have now talked to literally thousands and thousands of people around the world, and when I get the chance to ask someone a question, I almost always ask what they think good nutrition is all about. What does it mean to eat healthily? What do they call healthy food? Do they think the average Western diet is a healthy one? And then I ask them what they actually eat.

I am constantly amazed to hear two things. First, that everyone seems to know the basics of good nutrition. Just about everyone I meet recognizes the need to eat lots of veggies, fruits, nuts, wholegrains, legumes and seeds. And we all recognize that living only on sodas, pizzas and hotdogs is not the way to end up healthy. Not one person has said to me, 'Wow, Joe, I never realized that eating wholesome, fresh food from the farm was good for you. Thanks!'

What I found even more amazing is that everyone is pretty

much straightforward when it comes to the distance between what they think healthy eating is all about and what they actually eat. Everyone seems to know how important consuming fruits and veggies is, yet they go ahead and eat things that are loaded with chemicals and bad fats and too much sodium, all at their own peril.

I guess I shouldn't have been surprised. I did exactly the same for a long, long time. In Australia, when I was suffering from urticaria, I hired a nutritionist to cook fresh, wholesome meals for me every day. You know what I did after eating her meals? I ordered pizza and then hid the boxes in the garbage so she wouldn't find them. That's why I came up with the expression KIVDI, which stands for 'knowing it versus doing it'. How is it that we're not set free by being honest about our personal eating habits?

And that became my mission: to understand why, even when we know what's good for us, and even when we know what we should be doing, we don't do it. It shouldn't be that hard. But something is at work in our brains that causes us to make bad choices. Today I love fruits and vegetables. Yesterday I thought I loved hamburgers. But have you ever really savoured a fast-food hamburger? Try eating one cold, along with some cold fries. You know there's something wrong then. But I'm still tempted to eat cheeseburgers, and a lot more often than I'd like to admit.

I love my hard-won freedom from illness and the way that eating healthily makes me feel. Rebooters tell me they love being able to go on bike rides with their kids, or being able to buy regular-sized clothes, or how their joints don't ache any more, or how they no longer need to use a walker. Yet none of us are far from slipping back to where we were.

If you saw the movie *Fat, Sick & Nearly Dead*, you're familiar with Phil Staples, the truck driver who accepted my invitation to help him Reboot. His success was an inspiration to millions of viewers. But even Phil, after several years of healthy living, slipped back into his old habits and regained most of his weight (his full story is on page 29). Learning that Phil had a tough time of it, combined with my own struggle, had me searching for answers.

The big lessons

Why is it, then, that everyone seems to know the right thing to do when it comes to healthy eating, yet so few practise it? Even more importantly, why is it that so many people who have experienced the joy and liberation of healthy living end up sliding back? In this book we're going to break down the answers to that question and talk a lot about different tactics you can use to sustain your happy health. But first I want to look at the big picture.

If you ask me what are the big, overarching lessons I've learned over the last eight years, I would say that whether you succeed or not comes down to two relationships:

1 The relationship you have with yourself.
2 The relationship you have with plants.

The relationship you have with yourself – or the lack of one – is a huge key to understanding why we act the way we do. Most of us are way too critical of ourselves for a whole bunch of reasons. We have this inner voice that just beats us up. We look at ourselves in the mirror and, rather than thinking or saying something encouraging, we'll usually say something like, 'My God, what happened to you? You look terrible. Look at those bags under your eyes. Look at that belly. How old you look.' I know, because that was how I treated myself.

If you don't love and respect yourself, it's going to be a real challenge to sustain healthy habits. If you're like me, especially when you're faced with stress, you can quickly find yourself in the 'who really cares?' mode. That's when we put ourselves on hold. We don't exercise and we don't eat right because who really cares? What difference does it make if we're 20 pounds heavier?

Like many Rebooters, I've been a serial dieter. Some worked more than others, but no matter how successful, I'd return to my old ways and regain the weight. I would tell myself 'I have no willpower' or 'Diets don't work for me,' and then I'd give in, proving I had no willpower. I'd think of myself as a failure. Then I'd say, 'Who really cares anyway?'

Does that sound familiar? I think everyone has that inner voice, the one that's willing to accept defeat before you even get started. How to fix it? Start by answering the question of who really cares. That should be you, based on having a good relationship with yourself.

During the years after my Reboot journey began, I paid much more attention to this relationship, the one between Joe and Joe. I became conscious of it, and put effort and work into it. I learned to respect myself and the loving, nurturing, caring side of me. I always had respect for myself in business and in making money. But love affairs, with yourself or anyone else, are not about business. They're about looking in that mirror and, instead of saying, 'I'm a loser who can't succeed,' saying, 'It's OK. Today will be better. I'm taking a step in the right direction, and that belly – or whatever – is going to get better little by little. And you know what? I like those wrinkles, and the wisdom those grey hairs give me.' Yes, we've all got to be honest with ourselves and face what's in that mirror. But there is a big difference between self-honesty and being mean and hard on yourself.

The other big relationship is the one that people have – or rather don't have – with plants and the food that comes from them. They don't have the proper appreciation and respect for what Mother Nature provides. We are so besotted with processed foods that it's like we've lost our connection to the natural world. And believe me, I was one of those people. The last place where I wanted to spend any time in the supermarket was in the fresh produce section. Take me to the cakes, biscuits, frozen pizzas, deli meats, cheeses, pretzels and snacks, not to the greens.

But this relationship with Mother Nature, and with plants in particular, is also critical. Our understanding and knowledge of this food group is a supremely important relationship in our lives. We need to respect it, we need to honour it, we need to work at it, we need to embrace it – and we need to consume it.

When I meet people – and I've met tens of thousands in the last six years of my journey – I see individuals who are hurting, who are sick and tired, and many of them sick and tired of being sick and tired. And generally speaking, in every case, one or both of the two key relationships we're discussing is broken.

What I've learned since my Reboot is that these two relationships are crucial to health and happiness. Like any relationship, be it with family, friends or significant others, they need to be nurtured. We need to work on them and make them strong. You can't take yourself or plants for granted. You can go a few days or weeks with being a little bit absent, but you can't do that too often. Otherwise when we get stressed, and when the going gets rough, it becomes too easy to say, 'What's wrong with a cheeseburger and a chocolate shake? Who cares anyway? I'll have some veggies later.' But the longer 'later' gets, the more we forget how much we loved our veggies in the first place.

Taking action

So how do you tend to and care for the two major relationships in your life? How do you know it *and* do it?

The one with Mother Nature is the simpler of the two. As far as plants go, that's a lot of what the Reboot is about – learning how wonderful they are, what different plants can do for your physical and mental well-being.

The bottom line is that you've got to eat plants . . . lots of them. Don't take them for granted. Don't say I'll have some tomorrow because too many days without them will go by and you'll start to lose your love and appreciation of them. We'll look at how to eat after a Reboot, and the fact that there are many different 'diets' you can follow. The truth is, almost any one of them will work for you as long as it has a lot of plants.

Now, building a good relationship with yourself is harder. What does it even mean to have a good relationship with yourself?

I think it's about consciously making sure that when you are standing in front of the mirror, or going on your morning walk, or having a conversation with yourself on the train, you look for and stop the negative voice. I know all about this. There are many days when I get up and look in the mirror and think, 'Oh my God, look at you! You're a wreck, you've aged, you look puffy, you're fat. You no-hoper, you're a loser.' Not a great way to start your day, particularly if you have to go on a morning TV show to talk about your success and how much juicing has changed your life.

Instead of spiralling down into the abyss of self-pity, I need to remind myself that I am just like most people out there who are also in trouble. And that I'm going to try to do my best. True, I may not be where I want to be, but if I can make smarter choices today, I'll be one step closer.

That's being honest with myself, but it's also being kind. It's treating myself like I would treat a friend. And I reckon it's something that most of us need to remind ourselves to do.

So you need to take a good look at your relationship with yourself and at your relationship with the food that Mother Nature provides. Those are the basics, the two bookends. It's sounds simple – love yourself, love plants – but it's hard. Life likes to throw up hurdles – the bills that need to be paid, the endless nights on the road, a boss who constantly criticizes, a sick parent who needs care. These can knock us down and make us fail. But we can also successfully jump over them.

Seven steps to health and happiness

Here are seven things I've learned to keep me on my game, seven tools that can help you to sustain the healthy and happy life you deserve. We'll go into each one of these in much greater detail, but here's the menu for what to expect.

1 Change your relationship with food (don't abuse food).
One of the first things you need to do is to change how
you think about food, and how you use it in your life. A
huge amount of overeating is based on what we call
'emotional' eating, where you end up using food for something besides nutrition – perhaps as a way of dealing with
stress, or as a replacement for something that's missing
in your life, such as love or intimacy.

Emotional eating is very common, so you're not alone
in this. I'd say it was almost universal. That's what comfort
food is all about, using the experience of eating to take us
to happier times in our life. People also use food as a
punishment, after they have demonized it as bad. What
I've found is that you have to let go of all these inappro-
priate associations and uses of food, and get back to the
basics of regarding it as fuel, medicine and, of course,
something to enjoy.

2 Change your diet (eat the right stuff). There really is
something to the old adage that knowledge is power – the
power to make well-informed choices. Learning to eat the
right stuff means changing your diet, and that means
understanding the power of different plants.

I like to think of this as an extension of improving your
relationship with Mother Nature. Remember what I said
about how I never hung out in the produce section? Now
I love to check it out, to see what sort of magical fresh
plants a supermarket or wholefood store has in stock.
Once you go down that path, you'll find yourself reading
the labels, about this kind of Portobello mushroom, or
checking out that kind of Japanese aubergine (eggplant),
or fingering some red-stemmed chard you've never seen

before. The balance I like is the rainbow approach, where you try to get something red, green, yellow, orange and purple into your body every day.

3 **Change your habits (find a new groove).** After the shock of the Reboot, which is a quick way to reset your body and its relationship with food, you're going to return to the real world and all its pressures. So a lot of what you're going to deal with after the Reboot is how to change the behaviour you are used to – in other words, your basic food habits – while living in that real world.

Among the behavioural changes you'll have to make is, of course, modifying your diet so that it includes more nutrition from plants. But that means changing everything, from what you keep in your food cabinet at home, to how you serve meals to your family, and maybe even the places where you hang out during the day. In a world where seeing is eating, you might just have to change the route of that daily stroll past the bakery.

4 **Embrace community (get a little help from your friends).** I think that feeling down, depressed, alone or disconnected are dangerous times when it comes to actions that can hurt your health, be it abuse of alcohol, drugs, nicotine, caffeine, sugar, salt or fat. These times are when we start to feel that nothing matters, that no one cares, that we're losers and might as well trash the temple that is our body with a short-term fix of any of the above. But you can overcome these feelings of worthlessness with the help of others. You can seek professional help, but, more often than not, what you really need is the strength and joy that comes from community.

'But, Joe,' you say, 'I don't have a lot of friends. I've not had much luck with others. What can I do?' Here's another of the basic principles I live by: Lady Luck follows a person of action. What does that mean? You've just got to go out there and do it, whether it's joining an online community, or going to a gym, or becoming a local volunteer. By and large, people are friendly creatures. You'll be surprised by just how responsive the world is when you reach out. The worst punishment in prison (or anywhere, for that matter) is isolation. You can't succeed in life unless you join in.

5 **Maintain the machine (follow the upkeep manual).** 'We're only human.' How many times have I heard that? I think that's a kind of negative statement. I think it should be: 'Well, at least we're human.' Among other perks, it means we are given this fantastic thing called a body, the most complex organism in the universe – our brain alone has 100 billion nerve cells, with 100 trillion interconnections. It also has incredible systems for self-repair, which is more than you can say even for the most advanced machines out there.

Nevertheless, here's the deal: as with any piece of equipment that you cherish, you've got to maintain it. It needs upkeep. And that comes down to two things for your body: exercise and sleep. They're really two sides of the same coin. You can't exercise well without good sleep, and you can't sleep well unless you're getting good exercise. The more you pay attention to these two daily maintenance programmes, the easier it will be to sustain a positive, healthy lifestyle.

6 Practise mindfulness (chill out). After I ask people what they think healthy eating is all about, and then ask about their typical diets – only to find a wide chasm there – the next question is: Why? Why do you eat so much salt, sugar and bad fat? I get lots of different answers, including that they're too busy to eat right, or they don't like the taste of veggies, or it's not what everyone else is eating, or it's harder to find. But the biggest answer is that they're stressed out. And I know just what they're talking about. Put me under the gun and my knee-jerk reaction is to reach for Mother Sugar, not Mother Nature.

High on the list of how to sustain your health is dealing with personal stress. The sooner you figure this out, the better. Because odds are, unless you're a hermit living in a cave, your life is full of stress. Everyone's life is full of stress, from the head of government to the barista in your local coffee shop. Stress is a by-product of the modern world, and since you're probably not getting into a time machine tomorrow to head back to simpler times, you have to learn how to de-stress.

7 Respect yourself (stop beating yourself up). OK, this is kind of a repeat of the idea of improving your relationship with yourself. But I'm repeating it because, ultimately, nothing you do to improve your eating habits is going to work, or stick, or become a regular part of your life if you don't respect yourself.

It seems kind of obvious, but a lot of people aren't even aware of how mean they are to themselves, or how much they make a career out of putting themselves down. How are you ever going to improve your lifestyle and get to a healthy and happy place if you don't love yourself? Without self-love you're not going to care enough to make any changes, and most likely you'll be looking for ways to hurt yourself. Loving yourself is the foundation for all the actions I'm suggesting you take in this book; the good news is that with every step in the right direction, you'll love yourself just a little more.

That's it. After eight years of keeping my health together through ups and downs and enough stress to knock a bull off its feet, these are the seven things I think you need to sustain a happy, healthy life. The rest of this book is about these tools. Just remember that, besides the fact that there is no quick fix, no one silver bullet, there is also no single glove that fits all of us. It's why I don't like diets that say you've got to do this or that the 'right' way, or else. Like snowflakes and maple leaves, we all are unique, and we have to make these principles work for us as unique individuals.

PHIL'S STORY

Hardly a day goes by when I'm not asked about Phil Staples, the truck driver whose dramatic transformation was a big focus of the movie *Fat, Sick & Nearly Dead*. He was an important part of the film, an inspiration not only for millions of people who saw the movie, but for me as well. He was one of the first people to follow me into the world of Rebooting, and his success was contagious.

When I met Phil in 2007, at a truck stop in Winslow, Arizona, I felt like I was meeting my twin. I recognized the baggy oversize shirt trying to hide a huge round beachball stomach. I started talking to Phil and found out that he had the same auto-immune disease as me, urticaria. It was the first time I'd met anyone else with urticaria and I was half the world away from home.

Phil had been a long-haul driver for 25 years. Those years had not been kind to him. The gruelling hours behind the wheel, combined with the low-calibre nutrition that was typically his only option on the road, had resulted in massive weight gain and frequent flare-ups of urticaria that left his body aching and sore.

Phil's decision to reach out and ask for my help with a Reboot was documented in *Fat, Sick & Nearly Dead*. In fact, we extended the filming time by nearly a year to capture Phil's progress. And what we filmed was nearly miraculous.

Over the course of his 60-day Reboot, Phil lost nearly 7 stone (100 pounds). Over the subsequent year of living on a plant-based diet, he lost another 7 stone (100 pounds). And he became medication-free.

For several years Phil sustained his healthy gains. He got married and moved to Minnesota with a woman who was equally committed to a healthy, plant-based diet.

Then it all started to fall apart. Phil and his wife got divorced, and Phil began living with his nephew and some friends in what amounted to a student house. Eventually everyone moved away, and Phil found himself alone and depressed. It took more than a year, but in the end he regained all the weight he had lost – though, thank heaven, his urticaria did not return.

For Phil too the Reboot was the easy part. And while backsliding and gaining weight is always hard, for Phil it was particularly so. Here he was, the heart and soul of *Fat, Sick & Nearly Dead*, someone who had inspired unknown numbers of people to lose weight and get healthy, the 'if Phil could do it, I can do it' guy. But he couldn't sustain it. What does that mean for everyone else who followed his example? Is Phil a failure? Will they fail too? Or what if . . . Rebooting just doesn't work?

Now don't think for one moment that I believe any of those doubts. As I write this, Phil is getting back on track, and I know he will succeed. He will do it on his own timetable, not mine or my films. And I know that Rebooting works. But I also know it's not an end-all. You can't Reboot for life. It's the 'after the Reboot' that is the tricky part. The reason I made *Fat, Sick and Nearly Dead 2* and the reason for this book is to look at ways of avoiding a return to your old pre-Reboot lifestyle. How do you keep from backsliding?

I believe we have a lot to learn from Phil so I asked him to share his story of life after the Reboot.

Community, Connection and the Roller-coaster of Weight Gain

by Phil Staples

When I met Joe Cross I had been a cross-country truck driver for 25 years. I probably don't need to tell you what a truck driver's diet is like. It's the crappiest type of food you could ever get. The healthiest stuff you can find at a truck stop, at the smaller places, would be an apple or banana, or maybe the occasional refrigerated pickle. In the bigger restaurants you'll have a salad bar, but it's not always fresh and it'll have all sorts of yucky things in it like bacon bits and heavy dressings. Most everything from the kitchen will be comfort foods – burgers, steaks, chicken-fried steaks, macaroni and cheese, stuff like that. Not healthy at all.

I met Joe in November of 2007 at a truck stop in Winslow, Arizona – you know the Eagles' song? Here is this fairly fit guy approaching me with a funny accent, saying he's been drinking only juice, showing me pictures of himself 70 pounds [5 stone] heavier and he has urticaria? I didn't know what to think. I agreed to have a juice, and he gave me his card and said to call if I needed help. In April of the following year, just under six months later, I was miserable. I'd continued to gain weight, my urticaria was unbearable and I had trouble working. I didn't know what to do, so I took out his card and called him.

Joe called me back and said he'd help. I got time off work and moved into a little resort on a lake in Gull Point, Iowa. He coached me through a 30-day Reboot, and at the end of those 30 days I had lost 40 pounds [2½ stone]. I was already healthier too. When I started, my blood chemistry was what you'd expect for an overweight guy: high cholesterol, showing pre-diabetic markers and so forth. After 30 days, when I went back to the doctor, everything was normal. Before the Reboot, my heart had been enlarged; 30 days later my heart was darn near back to normal, just from juice fasting and walking. I did another 60 days, and at the end of 60 days I had lost 97 pounds [6½ stone]. I felt incredible.

When the Reboot was over I moved to a little town called Arnolds Park and started to work at a mom-and-pop healthfood store called The Market. Among my duties was teaching juicing classes. I was also working at the YMCA, going to their gym and using weights.

This was a great time for me. I joined a little church near where I lived. I had great friends there. One was a youth pastor and his wife. I had another friend who was a chef, an Israeli who was into a Middle Eastern diet. She was a very sweet lady who taught me to take on that kind of diet. She would make dishes for me, and would teach me in her store. It was a good life, going to church, doing things, helping the community. I had my juice classes three or four times a week.

I then met a woman and got married and moved to Minneapolis. The marriage was too quick: we got married three months after we met, stayed married for 13 months and then got divorced.

When the marriage ended, I called my brother and said come get me. I went back to Sheldon, where I was raised at the end of my childhood and where my parents still live. I was traumatized from the divorce, so I moved into a house with my nephew and his friends. It was good to have a lot of people around me. For a year or so I was still at a healthy weight. I had my nephew and his friends, my family nearby, and I was making good food decisions.

Every once in a while I would have some juice, but it wasn't like I was juicing on a regular basis. I was still trying to eat clean, but you can tell the difference in the way you feel. Even eating clean I would not feel as connected, not getting nearly as much out of it as when I was juicing.

Eventually I got left alone. My nephew got married and moved away, and everyone else left as well. What can I say? People leave because they have lives of their own.

After that it was just me and the house for the next six months. Between being alone and divorced, I didn't feel like the greatest person in the world. I felt like there must be something wrong with me. You just sit there and stew in the back of your mind, thinking of yourself that way. You start saying to yourself, 'I don't care, I don't care, I'm just going to do this or that.' And there is no one there to tell you any differently. So I ended up gaining weight. It took a while – well over a year – but in the end I gained back everything I had lost, some 200 pounds [14 stone].

I think a lot about what happened. Partly I think that people who go back to their old ways think they can always do a juice fast again. They think, 'I know how to do this and I can always do it again.' In the meantime, they get back into their old lifestyle, going out with friends and having big suppers with them and so forth. These are the 'good old' things that you think are OK because you can always get back into juicing.

Eventually, those 'good old' things keep adding up. I call them the 'OK tos' because you tell yourself it's 'OK to' eat crappy food because you can always go back to a Reboot. But eventually those 'OK tos' add up and shove you over the setback wall. The next thing you know, you're not paying attention and you're having a big old thick steak, or a big old cheeseburger, stuff like that. Eventually you're not even juicing, you're not eating healthy at all; you're back to having fast food and French fries.

Why this is the case, I don't know. I think a lot of people have food addictions and you have to treat them like drug addiction or alcoholism. I think some foods can also be addictive with the chemicals that are put in them. So the line that shouldn't be crossed is the first one, the first 'OK to'. It would be like an alcoholic going to a bar with friends and saying, 'Well, I can have just one, it's OK to.' You can't do that. Otherwise you just go back to your old ways.

But I also don't think it's as simple as that. I think that for most people there is a lot more to it. Rebooting is a really good plan to get the crap out of your diet, but you still have to get through the crap in your brain.

To be honest, for me it's a constant battle. It's between me and my brain. It's like I'm split somewhere down the middle. I've got this evil little voice in me going, 'Nobody cares about you, let's go have a burger.' And then I've got the me that says, 'I know better, so why are we doing this?'

What helps you get past that weird inner dialogue is having friends or people you can talk to. In fact, I would say it's critical, but I slipped away from it.

I eventually talked to Joe again. It was tough. I felt like I'd let him down. I didn't want him to know I wasn't doing well. But I can't tell you what a relief it was to finally raise my hand and say, 'Joe, I've gained weight, I'm struggling.' I started a second Reboot with Joe's help. He also sent Russ Kennedy, the behavioural psychologist who works with Reboot, to talk to me. It was really helpful having Russ there to help during my second Reboot. He was a good counsellor. I was free to talk to him and tell him anything. It was easy to get things off my chest and I was feeling better. And it went well in the beginning. I lost 50 pounds [2½ stone] – we'd been doing it a couple of months – and then I started cheating.

You see, what Joe couldn't give me was the community that I had back in Arnolds Park, or the intimacy I had when I was first married and living in Minneapolis. You have to create that for yourself.

So what I decided to do was to move here to this little town of Sheldon, to be with my folks, and with my brother and sister who live right nearby, and some of my old friends who are still here. Helping out my mom and my dad, who are now 80 and 75, is my volunteer work I guess you could say. My father just came home last month from the hospital, and he is still recovering from his operation.

After moving down here, I got myself a six-month pool membership and I go whenever I can. I'm on quite a few groups online, and reading all kinds of articles and recipes. People should do that too. It's not just Joe's website that has a lot of great information – the Internet is full of good articles and good advice for a healthy lifestyle. I've started eating vegetables again, and using a juicer my brother had, so I'm losing weight again.

If you ask me at this point what my best advice is, I would say that first you need to find someone to help you sustain a healthy life. I would say get as much support as possible, and not just through family. A lot of people have depression and similar problems in their lives. I'd say get medical support, but find your community too.

Get out into the world. If you're not going to a church, find one you like. Connect with friends, especially those who understand and support what you're going through. And volunteer. Help an old lady cross the street so you can get those good connections in your mind. Above all, don't just stay at home. You have to think of the house as a place to sleep. Otherwise it'll be a place to vegetate and rot and get fat again. You have to be outside and part of the world. It'll give right back to you.

Part II
THE SEVEN KEYS TO UNLOCK HEALTH

1

CHANGE YOUR RELATIONSHIP WITH FOOD (Don't Abuse Food)

In the previous chapter I talked about our two most important relationships. The first is our relationship with our self. The second is our relationship with plants, and with the nutrition we get from them. For the sake of brevity, I kept it simple. Just get more plants into your body.

That is good, straightforward advice, but our relationship with food in general, including plants, is a little more complicated than that. Not only is it a big part of our lives, it's also a very emotional one. And it's something we really need to understand because nothing you do when it comes to eating, or improving your diet, is going to last unless you change your relationship with food. If you don't have a good relationship with it, you will have a hard time with every other tip in this book.

When it comes to sustaining a healthy lifestyle, the key to lasting change is to understand the psychological side of eating – and that means, first and foremost, understanding your emotional relationship with food.

I cannot tell you how many people have said to me that they've tried every diet under the sun and that nothing works because they are 'emotional eaters'. Well, as psychologist Dr Russell Kennedy would say, everyone is an emotional eater. That is what makes us human. Think about it, Russ points out: from the day we are born, we start to associate food with comfort, community and love. Babies are nursed when they are hungry and when they need comforting.

As we grow older, we show our love through food and usually through unhealthy foods. Not many parents give their child broccoli when they want them to feel better after getting hurt; not many parents put candles on a pineapple instead of a birthday cake. I know several busy parents who insist on making their children's birthday cakes. Cooking special treats shows our love. What makes us feel better than Grandma baking us a batch of cupcakes, or serving us a plate of warm lasagne?

This bond of food goes beyond the immediate family. As a social species, we invest our shared eating experiences with huge emotional capital. For as long as we've been human, food has sewn together our social fabric. We celebrate just about everything with food, from formal meals for the whole tribe to ritualized social events for visiting heads of state. Almost every gathering we're part of – whether it's a date, a church social, a party, a wedding, even a funeral – involves food.

Eating is a fundamental part of our culture, and almost all eating has an emotional component. 'Our food has a lot to say about who we are as people,' says Dr Kennedy. 'It really makes us feel connected to our communities, our families and our cultures. It's a way that we show love to other people, to make or bring them food.'

Now there is nothing wrong with these emotional events.

They provide us with some of life's richest pleasures and most meaningful experiences. The problem comes when we start to use food's emotional connections as our primary tool to feel better, or to soothe ourselves. When this happens, our relationship with food becomes dysfunctional.

Comfort food is one of the best examples. We know that lots of people eat as a coping mechanism, especially in reaction to stress. It can also be a reaction to a more general feeling of unhappiness or loneliness. Since a lot of your relationship with food goes back to your childhood and to the foods you found comforting as a kid, eating can be a way of feeling safe, secure and cosy. It's an experience we're all familiar with.

When I was a kid, we didn't see my dad a lot during the week. He usually worked late and we were in bed by the time he came home. Friday nights my mother would drive us to the McDonald's near Manley Hospital in Sydney, where we'd meet Dad. Friday night was a ritual of family meals at McDonald's. Sunday evenings meant Catholic mass followed by 7.00 pm dinner at Hancourt Chinese Restaurant in Mosman. The maitre d's name was Herman and every dinner was the same – sizzling chicken, fried rice, honey corn. So our two nights out were Friday night McDonald's and Sunday Chinese.

Yes, I was hungry. And yes, I thought McDonald's and Chinese food tasted pretty good too. But the food also meant community to me. It was family time. It meant my parents' undivided attention, being silly in the back seat with my brothers and sister. So it's no coincidence that when I feel lonely, frustrated or stressed out, I really would like a burger, fries and a chocolate shake, or a big plate of fried rice.

I've also spoken publicly and written about how I was

frequently bullied in school. My mom and dad moved homes a lot. Dad was a doctor and Mom had a real talent for renovating homes and selling them. That meant us living in them, dealing with construction and then moving. This was great as every kid loves a building site, but as soon as it was all done and perfect, we'd move on to the next place. That meant we changed suburbs – and schools – a lot. Add to that our time in Columbus, Georgia, in the USA, where Dad went to further his orthopaedic training and I did third grade at St Anne's school.

With all this moving around, by the time I got to seventh grade I had been to six different schools. I was always the new kid on the block. And because I was big for my age, and kids were kids, I became a target. Lunches were lonely, I didn't have many friends, so of course I found another kind of friend. Sugar wouldn't let me down. It was always there to pick me up when I was having a bad day, and always there to celebrate with me when I was having a good day. And it wasn't just limited to school. After school there was nothing better than sitting down to watch *Get Smart*, *Gilligan's Island* and *The Brady Bunch* with a huge bowl of cereal and five or six spoonfuls of sugar. So what happens when I'm stressed, feeling like a loser or having a bad day? I want sugar! I want the couch, some ice cream and the TV! And, by the same token, what happens when I'm having a good day? Or when I'm celebrating my birthday with good friends? Well, I'd like some sugar then too because that's what I have when I'm having a good time.

Naturally, just what constitutes comfort food varies from person to person. Some of the tests that food researcher Professor Brian Wansink did at the Cornell Food and Brand Lab (where we visited with him for *Fat, Sick & Nearly*

Dead 2) found that comfort food for a woman is quite different from comfort food for a man. After surveying more than 1,000 people, his team found that for women, it's all about sweets – cookies, cakes and candy. It's about foods that represent freedom from cooking and cleaning. For men, it's more about pizza, pasta and meat, foods that their mothers may have cooked for them as children – foods that make them feel pampered and taken care of.[1] (So I guess when it comes to comfort food, you could say I'm in touch with my feminine side.)

Part of what you'll experience in a Reboot is a re-education of your taste buds and a new appreciation for plant-based foods. But your deep emotional links to food are just that – deep. It doesn't matter that I Rebooted, and it doesn't matter that I have a love of fruit and vegetables that I didn't have when I used to work on the Sydney stock exchange. My feeling today, pre-Reboot and post-Reboot, is the same. Sugar equals comfort, love and community.

It's seems obvious to me now that I am an emotional eater and sugar is my go-to food. But I didn't really make that connection between how I felt as a kid, what I ate then, and what I crave now as an adult until I was writing my first book, the companion to *Fat, Sick & Nearly Dead*. I was writing about my history with food and bingo! – it all became clear to me.

Since then I've been conscious of altering my relationship with food. An example of this is that New York City is not about pizza to me; NYC is definitely about juice. Don't ask me why, but I crave juice much more there than I do in Paris. I think it's because of what I do now, that I've made many new friends who've embraced a healthy lifestyle. I can't help but stay on track when I hang out with them. I've started to create a community and happy times that include juice, healthy foods and exercise. I've created new associations for 'comfort' food.

. We'll cover other 'doing' tips in the next few chapters, from what you should eat to how to keep from grabbing your go-to food and how to deal with stress in ways other than eating. But first you have to develop an awareness of your own comfort foods, and of the buttons you push with those foods. Awareness is the key here. You can't get a handle on your relationship with food until you become aware of it. Which is why, as an exercise at the end of this chapter, I'm going to ask you to write out a list of your favourite foods and why they're your favourites – including the happy memories you associate with them.

Food as a moral compass

I think one of the biggest mistakes we make with food is to use it as a moral compass. What I mean by that is how we give moral power to food, calling it good or bad, and turning each meal selection into a moral judgement. What usually follows is self-recrimination for eating 'bad' food, telling ourselves we're 'bad' people.

Let's get this straight: there is no such thing as good or bad food. Do you think that pizza is a bad food? Tell that to someone who is actually starving. To them, a slice of pizza is a slice of heaven. To someone with a health-threatening weight problem, however, a slice of pizza represents something very different.

Unless you're talking about something that is poisonous, food, in and of itself, is neither good nor bad. Some foods are more nutritious than others; some we like better than others, regardless of nutrient value.

Most of the people I've met, however, look at food as black or white: either good for you or bad for you. The problem is that when you eat 'bad' food, what you then say to yourself is: 'Because this is bad for me and I'm doing it anyway, I must be bad.' As someone who's been there and done that, I know this is not good for the spirit, or for the soul, or for the positivity we need to maintain a good relationship with ourselves. The next thing you know you start to punish yourself for being bad, and that can start a whole downward spiral.

Right here is where you change your relationship with food. Instead of beating yourself up because you just had some sweet or salty snack, give yourself a break. Make it a time to say, 'That was fun, that was great. I can't do that every day, but that was fun.' Then, if you want another one of those days, you can earn it. You can say, 'I'm going to try to focus on getting lots of nutrient-rich food for the next five or six days so that I can have another one of those days and really enjoy it.'

I think that's a much better way of thinking about it than what most of us do, which is scolding ourselves for having done something sinful. Believe me, I can still hear that voice: 'You're a loser for eating all of that. Tomorrow you get only water.' Instead of thinking how to punish ourselves, we should be focusing on getting things back in balance. The real question to ask is not why we over-indulged, but what's our game plan going forward? How are we going to get the more nutrient-dense foods into our system?

One of the reasons I'm not a big fan of 'diets' in the traditional sense of following a specific meal plan is that I think being told what foods are right and wrong is just another negative. As nutrition expert and author Dr Dean Ornish told us when we visited him, 'As soon as I tell somebody, "Eat this and never eat that, and always do this and never that," people just want to do the opposite. Talking to them in that way is not only unhelpful, it's actually often counterproductive.' Ornish likes to joke that the first dietary 'intervention' was when God told Adam and Eve not to eat the apple. 'That didn't work, and that was God talking,' he says, 'so we're not going to do better than that.'

A lot of people don't react well when you pass judgement on their food choices. And a strictly prescribed eating regime can have a negative effect, especially when people may be struggling to stick to a protocol that does not suit them. In the end, the diet police simply make you feel more down, more depressed, more like 'I'm not worthy', and that will steer you away from the nutrient-dense foods you need.

The bottom line is that there are a lot of food police out there telling us just what we should and should not eat. We don't need any more of those types to give us a hard time. You need to understand that food is not a fight between good and evil, and not the proxy for your moral struggles. Food is just food. It's how we choose to use it that makes all the difference. Most of the time it serves a nutritional function, and we love all those greens, reds and yellows, those salads, stir-fried veggies and lentil soups. Sometimes it serves a 'fun' function, like the joy you get out of eating an ice cream at the seaside. What you never want is food that's a tranquillizer for stress relief or a place to hide. With all due respect to the occasional nostalgic return to childhood, this is not how we should use food.

To be fair, most of the time when we eat for emotional reasons we are unconscious of the emotions. Sometimes we are not even aware of the eating itself. If, however, we are aware of what we're doing, if we are present in the moment, we can change our relationship with food from destructive to constructive.

Being aware

The most basic way to improve your relationship with food is awareness. If you are truly conscious of the food you are consuming, or are about to consume, this will make a huge impact on the way you eat.

This is true for a bunch of reasons. To begin with, a huge amount of overeating takes place when we're on what psychologist Kennedy calls 'autopilot'. The example he likes to give is when we're watching a big football game and we eat that bag of chips or crisps without thinking about it. Our attention is simply elsewhere, and we go on autopilot.

It's kind of like when you drive home while you're thinking about something else. Suddenly you find yourself in the driveway and don't remember getting there. Autopilot eating is like that, except that it has the added component of genetic behaviour, of our deep ancestral imperative to eat while the eating is good. We're programmed that if we don't eat the low-hanging fruit, someone else will.

It's quite amazing how much of our relationship with food goes back to our shared evolutionary past, and for good reason. Besides not getting killed by predators, eating was our top priority. Everything was built around hunting and gathering, and eating whenever we could. Taking a page from our primate relatives, sometimes we spent long hours eating forest fodder that was not as nutritionally dense as the food we have today. Just look at how much bamboo a giant panda eats: it gets through 26–84 pounds per day, so it's pretty much an all-day activity. That kind of eating requires going on autopilot.

Professor Wansink does a fantastic job of talking about this blank-out we have towards food in his book *Mindless Eating*. We'll look at some of his behavioural findings in the chapter on changing our habits about food. What's important here is how little attention we pay to eating, and how that results in us eating more than we think. Popcorn at the movies? In Wansink's experiments it didn't even matter if the popcorn was fresh. Give movie-goers a bigger tub of popcorn and they'll eat more of it anyway, like sleep-walkers.[2]

And it's not just our unconscious, mindless eating that calls for awareness. Taking another page from our evolutionary past, food companies use something that's come to be known as the 'bliss point' to scientifically take control of our brains and taste buds.

The bliss point concept comes to us from the famed American market researcher Howard Moskowitz, who helped food-makers understand that there is a maximum point for our appreciation of the 'big three' in food: sugar, fat and salt. Each played a key role in our nutritional survival – sugar gave us energy, fat could be stored, and salt kept our fluids in balance – so we crave these tastes. What manufacturers do is bring these nutrients to the fore, which makes the food they saturate taste so good.

We are practically helpless before this onslaught. Most processed foods are stripped of their natural fibre so the fat, salt and especially sugars go right to the bloodstream. You get a rush that makes you feel better right away. Never mind that you'll crash later from all that sugar, or that tomorrow your waistline will be that much larger. In the moment, where the reward is experienced, you feel better.

This is how food created in labs acts like a drug. Similar to heroin or alcohol, it gives you an immediate blast of pleasure. In our pre-civilized past salt, sugar and fat were rare, and we were ecstatic to get our hands on foods that contained them. Now we can get these things whenever we want, and we experience them with a drug-like pleasure. And, like a drug, foods high in the big three can become addictive. So, just as with drugs, you have to break that destructive relationship and replace it with a healthier one. Hugs not drugs. Or the runner's high instead of the heroin high.

These bliss point tricks used by the food manufacturers are not their only ploys. Besides engineering the flavour, they also engineer the appearance of food with artificial colouring, boost its appeal with bright packaging, and enhance its texture with processing.

The reason we're taken in by these ruses is that a lot of what and why we eat has to do with our brains and not our bellies. We are conditioned by visual cues that helped us survive – the bright colours of ripe fruit, for example, now hijacked by sweet-makers.

All of this shows just how important awareness is with food. When a magician performs a trick on stage, as long as we don't know the secret behind it, we're enthralled. We may not realize that the spaghetti sauce tastes so good because it is highly salted and sugared. Or that we buy one product instead of another because of artificial colouring. But once we are aware of it, we can make decisions on what we eat for the nutrition, not because of a gaudy show of taste, texture and appearance. The same goes for mindless eating; being aware of it can save you lots of calories.

The lost connection

I'm fairly sure that most vegans and animal lovers would not be happy with the opening scene of the movie *Last of the Mohicans*. In it, Daniel Day-Lewis, starring as Hawkeye, is running through the mountains with his Indian companions, just running and running. They are hunting a deer, which they eventually catch and kill with an arrow. However, what's remarkable from the perspective of our modern ways is how they bend over the slain animal and thank its spirit for providing them with sustenance. There is something organic and even spiritual about their relationship with the food that nature provides.

Contrast that to our modern relationship with food. We are disconnected from the source, from the natural relationship between Earth, sun and rain. Instead of grazing in the pasture, our livestock is raised in factory farms and the meat comes to us wrapped in plastic. Instead of getting our fruits and greens from local gardens and farms, they are packed and shipped in from gigantic plant factories, psychologically and physically distant.

In Michael Pollan's book about our love affair with certain plants, *The Botany of Desire,* he describes how potatoes are farmed today. They are spawned and raised in massive agribusiness complexes that produce monoculture Russet potatoes – the perfect size and shape for French fries – by using pumped-in petrochemical fertilizers, groundwater and a host of toxic bug and fungus sprays. One compelling anecdote is about an agri-biz potato farmer who would not feed his own family from his industrial produce, but instead grew a patch of potatoes in his backyard garden.[3]

Most of us, however, do not have a backyard garden. We are at the furthest end of the conveyor belt in our national food factory, divorced from the source. We no longer have a relationship with Mother Earth. The chemically imbued foodstuffs we eat, all re-engineered to taste better and last longer on the shelves, have become the norm.

One of the things that a Reboot does is reset our relationship with what we eat. Gone are all the cookies, crackers, snacks, sweets, cakes, crisps and so forth that have become such a large part of our diet. Instead there are only plants, the unadulterated fruits and veggies that come right out of the ground. And when we Reboot, a profound thing happens: our relationship with food changes. There is no longer a middleman processing it and altering it, embellishing it and pumping it with salts, sugars and preservatives. It's just us and the food itself. And in that Reboot process our body relearns what real food is all about. The connection is re-established, the original relationship renewed.

Consequently we learn to appreciate the real taste of food without the chemical and bliss point inputs. At first it's like trying to see the stars at night in a big city, where the man-made illuminations erase the natural light of the heavens. But as we turn down, or even off, the man-made lights, the sky begins to glow again, to come alive in all its natural complexity. We taste the real food again, and we re-establish our relationship with it.

Trust yourself with food

Another part of your relationship with food is what you think about it before you eat. Call it the spin. If someone says, 'Hey mate, this is great food,' you're going to give it a better rating than if someone says, 'Hey mate, this is terrible stuff here.'

Suggestibility is powerful stuff. Studies show how when we eat socially we tend to eat more than when we eat alone; we also eat in response to what others eat, and descriptions count for a lot. In one flamboyant experiment for *National Geographic* magazine, food writer Erik Trinidad set up a 'Roadkill Café' on the edge of a college campus, trying to see if people would try Possum Poppers, Iguana Lasagne or Blackened Beaver Tail. No takers, until he used speakers to amplify the sounds of sizzling and wafted the smell of grilled skirt steak into their faces, which got a couple of them to try the 'Beaver Tail'.[4] Likewise, Professor Wansink did experiments on suggestibility by serving people the same wine with different labels. If the label said it came from California instead of North Dakota, everyone said the wine tasted better.[5]

Part of changing your relationship with food is listening to yourself, not to someone else. How many of us have actually asked ourselves about the food we're eating, about which foods really work for us and which don't? How do you feel after you've eaten bread or spaghetti? How do you feel after you've eaten avocados or tomatoes?

The funny thing is that, when it comes to drinking, we all seem much more aware. If you have a cup of coffee, or a glass of wine, or a can of beer, you generally know how you'll feel afterwards. People have a really keen sense of it and will say, 'No, I can't have that glass of wine now' because they are certain of how they'll feel later.

How many of us are doing that with our foods and know how we'll feel? For myself, I know that if I avoid eating bread for a few days, I can smell things more intensely, I can see things more clearly, and I'll feel better, lighter. I have a sense of it because I have learned to pay great attention to the input and output of food for myself.

There is a funny little book called *How to Live One Hundred Years*, written by a nobleman named Luigi Cornaro, who lived in Venice from 1484 to 1566. (Yes, he was 102 when he died.) At that time, people believed that you had to eat more, especially meat, to stay strong as you aged. Instead, Cornaro spent years fiddling with his own diet until he had a 'perfect' balance of eggs, wine, vegetable soup, tomatoes, wholegrain bread and pure grape juice. The only time he faltered was when, in his eighties, relatives convinced him to eat more heartily, with more meat. He became violently ill and nearly died, only to return to health when he resumed his special diet.[6]

Cornaro is a great example of someone who listened to his own body, and who defied social pressures in order to establish his own highly aware relationship with food.

A new relationship

My Reboot gave me a new relationship with food and a brand new awareness of what I'm eating. My goal is to make that relationship instinctive, my new autopilot. My goal is to make nutritious choices when I don't have to think about it. That's the end game, where you will sit down in a restaurant and order the tomatoes and salad and white fish and fresh cucumbers, and order them not because you want to lose weight and be good, but because that's what you really want and what you really feel like eating.

When you think it over, it's a paradox. It's like having to make a judgement without judgement. On the one hand, we have to ensure that we get as much nutrient-dense food into our bodies as possible. On the other hand, we have to make sure that we don't go too crazy and become obsessive, and turn into a member of the food police. They are no fun to be around.

But we also want to be aware of our food in order to be thankful for it. Not forgetting about it in some mindless act of consumption. Not bolting it down fast on our way to somewhere else. Not being so disconnected from how food is prepared that we are no longer participants in the process.

Few things in this world are more important than our relationship with food. It's a long, long relationship, it's one we are going to have all our lives, and it's one we can't toss aside and replace with something else. That relationship does not have to be antagonistic or negative. It can and should be friendly and positive.

We should respect our food and where it comes from, and we should certainly be thankful for its abundance. The place where that relationship starts is respect for Mother Nature, and to honour the food for the health and nurturing it brings. Love those plants and you'll get the love right back.

FEELINGS ABOUT FOOD

Ready to delve into your emotional relationship with food?
Try this:

1 Make a list of foods that you associate with your childhood, especially the happy times. Think back on where
   your family went to dinner, the places you were excited
   to go. Try to remember the food your mother made for
   you when you were feeling ill or unhappy – the true
   comfort foods. Then see if these are 'problem' foods for
   you today.

2 Make a list of the foods you eat when you are at a party,
   or the ones you eat as a reward, or the ones you eat when
   you are under a lot of stress; often they are the same. See
   if these are the same as your childhood favourites. Then
   make a list of alternatives and try plugging these in when
   you are celebrating or soothing yourself.

3 Make a list of the meals you eat when you are consciously
   attempting to create a 'balanced meal' or to eat nutritiously.
   Are these foods you enjoy? If not, trying coming up with
   alternatives that provide the same nutrition but are foods
   that you like. Don't turn nutrition into a straitjacket.

4 Keep a food journal. Note not only what you are eating
   and when, but also how you feel prior to eating. Are you
   really hungry or are you feeling bored, anxious, lonely,
   happy?

'I've struggled with weight my entire life,' says Dr Carrie Diulus, a talented spinal surgeon who lives with her husband and two kids in Ohio. What annoys her the most, she says, is 'listening to a lot of people who've never struggled with weight loss talking about how easy it is to do. Just count calories, right? Sure, just eat more vegetables, right? Tell me that at 2am when I'm eating peanut butter and using a chocolate bar as the spoon.'

In her seesaw battle with weight gain, Carrie describes how she 'ballooned up' in college, putting on an extra 6¼ stone (90 pounds). She then lost that weight in medical school with a regime of intense exercise and calorie counting, only to regain 'a ton of weight' when she got pregnant in her thirties. She lost that weight, only to gain it back during her second pregnancy – when she also developed an uncommon medical disorder that produced too much fluid around her brain and impacted her vision.

About six months after giving birth, and still struggling with weight loss (though her medical condition improved with some shedding of pounds), a friend told her about the film *Fat, Sick & Nearly Dead*. 'In my lifetime I've been on every diet that exists,' she says, but this was a different approach, a shift from counting calories, fats or carbs to a lifestyle of eating unprocessed food, mostly plants. 'I bought a juicer the day after I saw the movie, and I went on a 42-day juice fast. I lost all of the weight and couldn't believe how amazing I felt.'

One big difference between the Reboot and her previous weight-loss regimes, says Carrie, is that she wasn't particularly healthy during her 'slim' phases; she was eating less but not necessarily eating nutritiously. 'For very few people is it really just about food or just about exercise. It's not just about the laws of thermodynamics. It's about feeding yourself the right nutrients.'

Even after her Reboot, however, Carrie found herself slipping back into bad habits. 'I kept most of the weight off, but then life got very stressful,' she says. Before too long, with stress at work combining with the stress of raising small children, she found herself losing sleep and turning to carbohydrates and junk food for relief. 'I was trying to medicate with food,' she says. 'Before I knew it I'd gained about 30 pounds [over 2 stone] from where I wanted to be.'

Rather than surrender, Carrie got back on the horse and returned to a healthy diet and lifestyle – motivated in part, she says, by some stern warnings from her own doctor that she was headed towards Type 2 Diabetes. 'I was motivated by the labs [test results] and motivated to prove I could cure myself to the docs that wanted to put me on meds . . . I don't want to end up diabetic.'

Besides paying more attention to a plant-based diet, Carrie also reached out for help from colleagues and friends, including her husband, to ask for their support in her struggle. Most importantly, however, she addressed one critical problem – inadequate sleep. 'When life got really stressful, I wasn't sleeping well,' she says. From her own studies of biochemistry, Carrie knew this meant her body was generating more cortisol, a stress hormone that leads to a host of problems if you produce too much, including weight gain.

So her focus was on relaxation. 'We all have stress, but how we manage it is what makes the difference. I had to get back on top of my sleep, so I had to get back into the concept of stress reduction, with meditation and exercise,' she says. Figuring out how to get back on track is 'a matter of taking a personal inventory. Where do you need the most work? Then you set up the plan from there . . . For me, once I got my stress under control, the food part came easier. I didn't have to pay as much attention to avoiding junk food because I didn't crave those things as much.'

The main thing, says Carrie, is not to panic – and to understand that you are human. 'Life is going to happen, and some factors you can't change. You have to figure out what you can do. My goal isn't about the number on the scale, it is about taking care of my own health and being an example to my kids and my patients.'

2

CHANGE YOUR DIET
(Eat the Right Stuff)

I like to keep it simple. For me, eating healthily means consuming lots of fruits and veggies – eating them, blending them and juicing them. I feel that eating healthily is all about balance, and about getting a lot more plants – and that means fruits, vegetables, nuts, beans and seeds – into your system.

There are really only three sources of energy for us, and by that I mean food. You can eat food from plants, food from animals or processed food. For most of our human existence we've had just two choices: plants or animals. We were great with that because we like having just two choices: black or white, hot or cold, friend or foe. Then came processed foods, the stuff you typically find in the centre of the super-market, filled with preservatives, artificial flavours, and our bliss point trio of sugar, salt and fat (and not the good kind of fat, either). These processed foods weren't even available a century ago, but today they're everywhere, a blinding array of choices that tempt us with empty calories.

People ask me, 'Joe, do you think eating McDonald's or food from a quick-service restaurant (QSR) is bad for you?'

To answer this question I think we need to bring in some perspective. If you go to McDonalds or a QSR once or twice a month but are eating a tremendous amount of plant food the rest of the time, I find it difficult to see a problem with those infrequent visits. The problem is when fat or processed food is all or most of what you are eating. In my view it's what you're leaving out that is dangerous to your health. I think this philosophy enables us to go to the football game or that special event and really enjoy the hotdog or piece of cake with a smile on our face and – better yet – free of guilt.

Unfortunately, this balance/moderation is not happening for most of us. Research shows that the Standard American Diet (SAD) derives 60 per cent of its calories from processed foods, 33 per cent from animal sources, 2 per cent from potatoes/french fries and just 5 per cent from plants, including beans, nuts and seeds, fruits, vegetables and wholegrains. [1] And, unfortunately, the rest of the world seems to be following suit.

One of the big benefits in my life now is that I get to talk and meet really clever and interesting people who have been studying and researching nutrition for most of their lives. It's a complicated subject, but here, in very simple terms, is what they taught me.

When we talk about nutrients we have two categories: macro (large) and micro (small) nutrients. Macronutrients are the ones we've all heard about – protein, carbohydrates and fat. One way to look at these guys is that they're the building blocks of energy, as well as all of the body's tissues and organs. Micronutrients, meanwhile, are vitamins, minerals, phytochemicals, zoochemicals, certain acids (e.g. phynolic), and tens of thousands more trace chemicals. The way I like to think about this group is in the form of tools or implements. These are needed for the body to process and transform the macronutrients.

So instead of thinking about the food we eat as just energy, I like to think about the food we eat as energy plus a toolkit. The energy part is self-explanatory, but with the toolkit, think about it this way: our cells need certain molecules, especially ones they can't make themselves, to function at optimal levels. Vitamins B, C and D, and minerals such as iron and zinc – these won't give us the energy to run a marathon. But they will give us the saws, hammers, nails and glue our cells require to transform macronutrients into the energy to power our marathon run. When we're missing tools in this kit, we also open ourselves up to disease, since we can't build as strong an immune system.

So where do we find micronutrients? We find them mostly in plant foods. If you want to get technical, you find some zoochemicals in animal products, but the majority of them are found in plant foods. Macronutrients are found in all foods – processed, animal and plant. So when you look at the Standard American Diet we can calculate that out of every 20 calories consumed, 19 are loaded up with energy (macronutrients) and just 1 calorie contains the kit (micronutrients) that our cells need to function at their best.

What's happening is that we are eating calories devoid of nutrition. All the wonderful things that Mother Nature provides through plants – hundreds of micronutrients that our cells need to function properly – are just no longer there. Once our bodies process all the sugar, fat and salt we've just devoured, we immediately get hungry again because all the cells in our bodies are screaming for nutrition. And all those extra calories we just processed go into the storage system we call fat.

I used to order lots of my meals from the McDonald's drive-through. It was great because I didn't even have to get out of the car. I would order a Big Mac, a Quarter Pounder with cheese, a regular cheeseburger, a large portion of fries, a chocolate sundae, a chocolate shake and a Diet Coke. (I don't know why I ordered the Diet Coke; I guess I just liked the way it tasted.) The server at the window would say, 'You've got the family at home, huh?' and I'd say, 'Yup,' then drive off, find a parking space and wolf down the whole lot in ten minutes. And surprise, surprise – a couple of hours later I was hungry again.

When I was planning my first Reboot in search of a way to cure myself, I realized that this energy – this food – that I was putting into my body wasn't the right stuff. Everything I was eating was white or brown or black. I was eating food so far removed from nature that it didn't have any colour. It was food that had been stripped, bleached, processed or deep-fried, then re-packaged and infused with artificial colours and flavours. The food had energy but few nutrients.

So when I started my Reboot, after having tried every other yo-yo diet in the book, I wanted to cut to the source. I thought, what if I ate only food that was made by Mother Nature? What if I consumed only fruits, veggies, nuts, seeds and beans? And what if I started out by drinking only fruits and veggies, getting concentrated nutrients? Could I cure myself? Could I get off all the medications for my auto-immune disease?

What I'd already learned from my research was that 70 per cent of diseases are caused by lifestyle choices.[2] That still strikes me as just unbelievable, but you'll find that most doctors agree with that figure. And what are the lifestyle choices that lead to these deadly illnesses? They are what we eat, what we drink, whether we smoke or not, how much (or little) we exercise, how much we sleep, how we deal with stress, and how much love and intimacy we have in our life. Show me an overweight person who drinks loads of alcohol, smokes a lot, never exercises and lives with lots of stress, and I'll show you someone who will not be able to ignore the biological laws of cause and effect.

The research out there backs me up in spades. There are studies galore that show how eating more fruits and veggies reduces the risk of diabetes,[3] how eating too much salt leads to heart attacks,[4] how people with diets high in meat die younger than people with diets high in vegetables[5] – even how people who eat more vegetables and fruits are more optimistic, curious and positive.[6]

Probably the most important of these studies came out just this year, a British study of the eating habits of 65,000 people, which showed that those who consume seven servings of vegetables and fruit a day reduce their risk of death – regardless of other habits – by 42 per cent. If you just eat one or two veggies a day, your risk of death drops by 14 per cent; that increases to 29 per cent if you go to three or four portions; and by 36 per cent if you go to five or six. Seven seems to be the magic number.[7]

Just look at the Japanese, who have a much higher intake of fruits and vegetables than the typical Western citizen, and who consume much less sugar. As a nation, only the residents of tiny Monaco have a longer average lifespan.[8] The Japanese also have a much lower incidence of heart disease than the USA, UK, Australia and New Zealand, and tend to stay healthier longer as they get older (they would do even better if they didn't have so much salt in their diet).[9] In virtually every population where people live longer and healthier lives their diet tends to be plant-based.

By the way, you'll notice that what I'm talking about here is health, not weight loss. That is an important way to think about diet. If you eat for health, the weight is going to come off. Weight is just a by-product of an unhealthy diet. If you replace a lot of those processed foods you consume with nutrient-rich plants, you're not going to be hungry all the time, so you'll eat less sugar, salt and fat. Eating healthy is much more about eating the right stuff than about eating less.

I used to look at vegetables just as decorations on my plate, or something I plucked off my hamburger. Now I think of plants as the miracle of life, the way that life on Earth figured out how to get energy directly from the sun. So I look at plants as harnessed sunlight. Sometimes they're green, sometimes purple, red, yellow or orange. These are the colours of plants, and we should try to get them all into our diet because we want to ingest that entire rainbow of nutrition. Remember, the reason we see colours is not so we can enjoy colour TV. Our ability to see colours is because of fruits and vegetables. We're built to recognize the colours of what we can eat so we can easily find food. Colourful fruits and vegetables therefore get top billing. So take the hint from Mother Nature and go for the rainbow.

Working it out

Practically speaking, there are two parts to healthy eating: finding a diet that works for you, and then sticking to it. What we're looking at here is how to find a diet that suits you; the rest of this book deals with how to sustain that way of eating.

One of the reasons I think juice-only Reboots tend to work for people is that juicing is easy. It's very black and white. The only decision you need to make is whether to include the peel on the lemon or the kiwi. If you've tried other diets – from calorie counting to South Beach and Atkins – you know you face myriad temptations throughout your day. Couldn't you have just a little cheese on the salad? Or how about a bit of bacon? That won't completely blow your diet, and you were so good at breakfast and lunch, right?

With juicing it's simple. All plants. You can't juice cheese or bacon. And there is no cap on the amount of juice you can drink. The more the merrier.

Moreover, Rebooting is just what it sounds like, a period of time to restart your body's relationship with Mother Nature. I would never suggest – nor could I ever live with – a diet of juice alone. Sooner or later you have to come back to solid foods, and integrate your intake of plants with a way of eating that you can sustain over the years. That, by the way, is the downfall of most diets: they are so restrictive that they feel like prisons. People break out and then go wild. I know because that's just what I did. Hey Joe, you lost weight on that diet? Great, let's reward you with a wild weekend of pizza and beer!

It seems that most Rebooted people, even those who did just a short one, finish with a newly found love of fruits and veggies. And the longer the Reboot, the more committed they are to eating healthily after their Reboot. But what does 'eating healthily' really mean?

Walk through the grocery store aisles and you'll see plenty of packaging that's labelled fat-free, sugar-free, gluten-free, 100 per cent natural, antibiotic-free, organic, and so forth. Does that mean these are all healthy options? You probably have friends telling you how great they feel after giving up wheat, or how unhealthy dairy is. Does eating healthily mean you need to give up eating ice cream for good?

Again, let's go back to the basics. It's not so much what you eat that makes you unhealthy. It's what you don't eat – the stuff you're missing. Remember what the father of medicine, Hippocrates, said: 'Let food be thy medicine and let medicine be thy food.' If you don't take your medicine – your plants – you can't be healed. But that doesn't mean you have to live in a plant-based straitjacket.

Since I finished my first Reboot seven years ago, I still haven't had coffee, alcohol or nicotine, and I still haven't had Coca-Cola. But I have had chocolate, and chocolate ice cream, and fish, and after four years I started to eat meat again, mostly white meat and very occasionally red meat.

As I've said, I'm not vegan, which can often surprise people, given my love of fruits and veggies. The majority of my diet today is from plants. I try to stay away from processed food – anything with a label listing lots of chemicals and additives. If I'm going to have tomato sauce, for example, I'd like it to be homemade, not from a can. I do love my sushi and a good sandwich, but in the past seven years the number of times I've eaten food from a quick-service restaurant I can count on one hand.

I have two meals a day that come predominantly from plants, and then one – usually dinner – that includes animal products. So I'll have juice for breakfast, or maybe a fruit salad, and sometimes eggs. For lunch it's almost always a salad, where you can throw in all sorts of interesting stuff, and then for dinner maybe some fish or lean chicken, along with veggies and wholegrains. Every now and then, maybe once a week, I'll reward myself with some food from what

I call the 'fun' part of town, usually in the form of chocolate ice cream. Am I perfect? No. Do I find myself too often in the 'fun' part of town when life gets a little unbalanced? Yes. But when I start to gain weight, when I start to feel low on energy and foggy-headed, it's because I've gone too far astray. It's because I'm not doing what I know is right for me. KIVDI. Knowing it versus doing it.

Looking at the Reboot team, I see that we have every type of eater – vegan, vegetarian, paleo, gluten-free, omnivore; some drink alcohol, some don't; some drink coffee, some drink soda. If you were to look at them, you would have no idea who ate what. You can't tell by their size, their energy level or the tone of their skin. What they have in common is that they are all a pretty healthy lot, even those with chronic illnesses (they are managing these through their diets). And they all drink a lot of juice. Yes, our company parties have alcohol, and usually someone is challenged to come up with a juice concoction that's also a great mocktail. You won't see processed or packaged food on the Reboot kitchen counter, but you might see some gluten-free or vegan cake, or maybe a raw dessert. So yes, we do all have sugar!

What's my point with this? I believe that the best diet for you is exactly that – for you. I don't dictate that my employees follow my diet. What's best for me might not be what is best for them. I love bread, but when I eat it, I tend to feel bloated, yet still want more. So I try hard to limit my consumption. You might not have any issues with bread, but I do. You might be lactose-intolerant, so you'll do better on a diet that eliminates dairy. I don't have that issue, so I can eat my ice cream once in a while. And within any of the broad diet categories, there's room for a lot of individual variations to eat plants – lots of them!

Now my very good friend Dr Joel Fuhrman, author of *The End of Dieting* and the father of the movement towards nutrient density, advocates a 100 per cent plant-powered diet. When pressed, he is actually fine with a tiny proportion (about 10 per cent) of animal products. But the problem Dr Fuhrman notes is that for many people moderation won't do the trick, and that they're never going to permanently kick their cravings unless they swear off sugary and processed foods altogether. 'Once you have gone through a Reboot, you've gone through all the withdrawal, and you're not craving the rich foods that are destroying your health,' he says. 'If you go back to eating them again, especially if you have food addictions, it makes self-control more difficult. It perpetuates the foods causing the problem.'

Food triggers and addiction, both of which we address in this book, are certainly problems for many people. When you are deciding what diet to follow, you need to be honest with yourself. Will moderation work? Did you get to your unhealthy state because you are addicted to salt, fat and sugar? Do you do better with hard and fast rules? What is the approach that will allow you to consume a high proportion of plants and stay healthy?

What are your eating options to begin with? We've provided definitions of some of the most common diets. You'll find more diet books and cookbooks for these specific diets than you can ever read. If you decide you want to learn more, just head to your local library or bookstore. We've also included a list of some of our favourites in the Further Information section (see page 231).

Diets Defined

Dairy-free: Excludes milk from cows, sheep and goats, and any products that contain them, including cheese and yogurt. Apart from the plant-based diet, many other diets are also dairy-free.

Gluten-free (GF): Eliminates foods containing gluten, a protein composite found in wheat (including kamut and spelt), barley, rye and triticale. Gluten can cause digestive problems in some people.

Macrobiotic: Focuses on eating grains as the main staple, in addition to local vegetables, and avoiding highly processed or refined foods and most animal products.

Paleo: Takes its cues from how the Paleolithic caveman ate. If it wasn't on the plate 10,000 years ago, it's not likely to be in the paleo diet. Anything that requires agriculture or farm animals is out. Anything we could hunt or find, including meat, fish, nuts, leafy greens, fruits and seeds, are in. This means a paleo diet is also dairy-free and gluten-free.

Pescatarian: Similar to a vegetarian diet, but includes fish too.

Plant-based: High in vegan foods (fruits, veggies and wholegrains, such as rice, quinoa and barley) but not limited to them. The term can cause confusion as some people use 'plant-based' to refer to a vegan diet. I call veganism a 'whole plant diet'.

Raw: Contains only uncooked and unprocessed foods. People who follow a raw diet eat fruits, vegetables, nuts and some grains. This is rather like the human diet before fire was discovered.

Vegan: Consists only of plants. Allows no animal flesh (red meat, poultry or fish), or any products that have come from an animal, such as eggs, milk and butter.

Vegetarian: Allows no meat, poultry or fish, but may include eggs and dairy products.

At Reboot with Joe we analysed over 10 of the recommended government and research institute diets: those from the US Department of Agriculture (USDA), Cornell University, Harvard University and the UK's National Health Service (NHS), as well as popular plans such as Atkins, South Beach and the Palaeolithic. Here's what they all had in common: *eat mostly plants*. Even the diets that had the least amount of plants recommended a minimum of 35 per cent plants (by weight). So pick a diet high in plants and you can't go wrong.

In figuring out what diet is best for you it is important to pay attention to the following three things.

1 Food sensitivities

Many people have food sensitivities that may include allergies or health conditions such as coeliac disease (an intolerance of gluten). Obviously, if you have food allergies or health conditions that are aggravated by certain foods, these will influence your diet. People with nut allergies may have a hard time with a raw diet as it relies heavily on nuts.

2 Triggers

Some food we eat just because it tastes good and makes us happy. There is nothing wrong with these 'comfort' foods, so long as they remain a small part of your diet. There are certain foods, however, that act as triggers for what amounts to compulsive eating. For example, you might not be able to eat a bowl of chocolate ice cream because if you do, you will polish off the whole carton. Some people call this food addiction, and there is even evidence now that it is genetic.

Regardless, we all have our trigger foods. These are foods you have to avoid, and the sooner you figure them out, the better. I don't drink alcohol because it goes hand-in-hand with smoking for me. I may have a beer or glass of wine someday, but for now I think the temptation to smoke would be too great. The reason I don't drink cola is because I can't have just one. I love the stuff, so sugary and full of caffeine. But I haven't had one in seven years because I know if I do, I won't stop.

3 Ethics

For many vegetarians and vegans, their adopted diet is as much an ethical choice as it is a health one. How do you feel about consuming animals? Are you OK with the concept of eating another living creature? How do you feel about the environmental impact of livestock? Among other things, it takes much more energy to produce animal food than plant food. In fact, only 55 per cent of the world's crop calories feed people directly; more than a third goes to feeding livestock (the rest is used for synthetic fuels and industrial products). Beef is the worst culprit; besides producing huge amounts of methane gas, the world's 1.5 billion cows give us only 3 calories of energy for every 100 calories of grain used to feed them.[10]

These are some of the things to think about when it comes to figuring out the best diet for you – including the ethical considerations. Yes, I consume animals. I have more fish than meat, and keep meat to a small part of my diet. I try to stick to grass-fed, antibiotic-free, free-range and locally raised meat. Not only is it healthier for me, it's healthier for the environment.

Your diet may also change over time. During the filming of *Fat, Sick & Nearly Dead*, I drank fresh juice for 60 days. I followed that by three months of consuming only whole-plant foods. I didn't eat meat for the first four years, but then I added a little meat every so often because I listened to my body and it felt right.

What's important to know is whether your diet is changing because you are changing (for the better!) or because of an outside influence (see Chapter 3 on food habits). Are you fully in control of the food choices you are making? Are you the master of what you eat? Or are you letting lack of sleep, loneliness, stress or something else make the choice for you?

And don't fool yourself. You can make unhealthy choices within your healthy diet. I meet vegetarians who spend a lot of time in the land of beige foods – bread, cheese and pasta. They may be vegetarians, but their diet is often no better than the Standard American Diet. You can get just as much sugar from a chocolate vegan shake as from regular ice cream.

At the end of this book, I've included a three-week meal plan and recipes for my diet. This is how I strive to eat. Use it for inspiration, but adapt it as you see fit. Come up with your own three-week plan for healthy eating and use it as a touchstone, following it to the letter at least once, and you'll have a greater understanding of how you want to eat – plus the 'doing' will be easier.

Even with the best plan, however, the odds are that you'll go off track. You'll find yourself making unhealthy choices. The rest of this book deals with tools to help keep you on the path you have chosen.

Ready to figure out your optimal diet? Try the following:

1 **Try an elimination diet.** During an elimination diet you remove a specific food from your diet for 15 days, then reintroduce it. If you suspect that you are lactose intolerant, for example, eliminate any dairy from your diet for 15 days. Then add it back in its whole form by drinking a glass of milk. How do you feel? You should notice a difference if dairy is an issue for you – either better by the end of those 15 days without it, or not as great when you add dairy back in. If you are allergic to milk, you should notice an immediate effect. A Reboot works really well as an elimination diet. After a 15-day or longer Reboot, slowly introduce foods back into your diet one at a time and note the effect of each.

2 **Keep a food diary.** Keeping a food diary is a terrific tool for understanding how different diets affect you, and what foods work best for you. Keep a diary of what you eat for two weeks, entering every single thing (and how much of it) you consume. At the same time, keep track of how you feel, especially after you eat. Look for correlations between food and how you feel. Do you notice that you have indigestion after consuming dairy? Do you get a headache every time you have red wine? It's important to consume a variety of foods during the time you keep a food diary. If you have bread, cheese and wine every day, you will not be able to correlate how you react to specific foods.

3 **Consider the ethical issues.** Think what you care about in terms of sourcing food. Do you care where it comes from, how it is grown, what it costs, its availability? Do any of these considerations factor into your choices?

4 **Identify the foods that you eat all the time.** Do you have soda one or more times a day? Do you crave chips and dips and eat them almost daily? Are you able to eat them in moderation? Leave them out of your diet for two weeks and see how you feel.

A changing relationship with food
Ciruu Kiniti

Whatever questions you put to attorney Ciruu Kiniti, just don't ask her when she plans to return to a 'normal' diet.

'People ask me when am I getting back to normal eating. I get this a lot. What do they think normal is? For me this is normal,' she says. 'If you can get all the nutrition you need into your body, then that is normal.'

As a resident of Kenya's capital city of Nairobi, Ciruu comes from a culture where eating is central to social interaction. 'It's a social thing. It brings us together. Being in that position, I'm asked every time, why aren't you eating? And people here have not heard of juicing. They think you're not being healthy. My first big lecture came from my dad. He said, "If you want to lose weight, do it the right way!"'

But the 'right way' had never worked before. So when Ciruu decided to Reboot – after watching *Fat, Sick & Nearly Dead* 'three or four times, so I could really download it into my spirit' – she Rebooted with stubborn determination.

'The decision to do this was for myself. I needed to change,' she says. 'Still, there were social functions, dinners to go to, weddings to attend. I would come carrying my juice and people would laugh. I went to a big family dinner at a restaurant and I just asked the waiter for a glass. They couldn't believe it.'

In the end, Ciruu juiced for 100 days and lost more than 4 stone (60 pounds), and her family and friends became her biggest support group. 'I had to explain myself at first. They acted like I was in a cult of some kind. Now people can see that I am much healthier than I was; they have seen my change, and they hold me to it. I hold myself to it for others too, so I must keep to this for them. Community really makes me do it,' she says. 'My dad is today my number one fan.

He is very proud of me, very proud, and has me come and talk to the ladies in his town.'

Like other viewers of *Fat, Sick & Nearly Dead 2*, Ciruu saw what happened to Phil Staples. 'I really sympathize,' she says. 'Without that support, without family and people around you that you can talk to, you go back very quickly and the pounds will just pile up. Community is key and very central.' Ciruu is also part of an online juicing group, and has received so many email queries about juicing that she had to compose a 'Hi All!' response that includes an explanation of juicing, links to the *Fat, Sick & Nearly Dead* site and her support group, and some basic recipes.

Because she juiced for 100 days, Ciruu says that she also experienced what she calls 'permanent changes' in her body's relationship with food. Among other things, her taste for red meat has disappeared. 'I don't know if there is such a thing as an addiction to red meat, but there was for me. In Kenya we have something called *nyama choma*, which is like a barbecue, and I did a lot of that,' she says. 'Now I can't eat red meat. I can't even look at it.'

Ciruu currently gets her protein from beans and fish, sometimes chicken. But she eats these – in much smaller portions – only at night, keeping to juice and salads during the day. 'I lean towards the food that talks to me now. This is really a complete transformation.' Her one weakness, she says, remains cookies. 'I'm not perfect. The vice I have left in my life is ginger cookies. That is one vice I can't shake.'

What has changed, she says, is that she doesn't 'demonize' her treats any longer. 'I'm fine with going to that side of the street, as long as I pull myself back before I go over all the way. I tell myself, I'm not where I was before. I'm in control now. I never walked before, and now I can walk those calories off.'

Before her Reboot, Ciruu says she never exercised. Now

she walks an hour a day and jogs a few times a week. 'Before the fast I couldn't walk and talk at the same time. I had to choose one or the other. I would literally have to stop and talk, or else just walk in silence. Now I can run and talk.'

It's all part of what Ciruu says is a new way of life. 'This is a brand new person. Everything about me has changed. My mind is sharper. I sleep better and dress better and I have a better self-esteem,' she says. 'This is not a fad, it's not a diet. It's something that changes your approach to how you look at food . . . I still juice every day. It's like drinking water. It's become part of my life. It's me now.'

3
CHANGE YOUR HABITS ABOUT FOOD
(Find a New Groove)

I call the distance between your hand and your mouth 'the last two feet of freedom'. No matter what any television ad seduces you with, or what anybody puts in front of your face, or what anybody suggests you eat, what you actually eat is still your choice, unless you've been strapped down and force-fed. In the end, no one is making you lift your hand from the plate to your mouth.

The problem is that most of us don't always make healthy choices. As I've already said, just because you know the right thing to do doesn't mean you're going to do it. KIVDI.

Before we start beating ourselves up, however, I'd like to point out that the cards are stacked against us. The number of temptations we face on a daily basis is mind-blowing. There is a giant marketing machine out there trying to get us to eat more all the time. When I drive past a billboard that says, here, have a refreshing fizzy drink, suddenly I want a Coke. I didn't want one two minutes earlier, but now it's back in my head.

Let's be honest here. We are all creatures of habit and conditioning. The physiologist Ivan Pavlov, who conditioned dogs to salivate when he rang a bell, got it right. We learn to do things in a certain way, and then those behaviours become ingrained and automatic. They become habits and are hard to break. According to scientists, more than 40 per cent of the actions we perform each day are driven by habit rather than conscious decision-making. The good news is that they can be changed, especially if you employ the right strategies.

A history of habits

We develop habits because they serve a very useful function. If we had to reinvent ourselves every day, life would be chaos. Habits are really nothing more than things we've learned to do by repetition, for the sake of efficiency. If you want to do something well without thinking about it – like riding a bike, or throwing a spear, or speaking a language – it had better become a habit.

Naturally enough, when it comes to food we all have habits as well. You probably buy the same brand and type of cereal or crackers over and over. You walk down the grocery aisle and pick up the same coloured box every time. It's easier than looking at the ingredients and trying to determine which one you'll like best, or which one is the best for you.

Like most habits, our eating routines are well-worn patterns of behaviour that also become a comfortable, well-worn path. If you're used to grabbing a fizzy drink and a bag of snacks when you get home after work or school, that habit becomes a ritual of comfort, a pleasure you can look forward to and rely on.

To give you an example of how strong a habit can be, when I was on my 60-day Reboot across the USA, I'd check into a motel and would quite often find myself opening up the mini-bar to have a look inside. I'd do this even though I was on, say, day 45 of just juice. I was so conditioned from the previous 20 years of my adult life that it was a default action to open the mini-bar and look for the Kit-Kat, the Mars Bar or the Snickers. Basically it was autopilot.

Why habits are so tough to break or change comes down to brain chemistry. For every experience we go through, there is a change in our brain's electrochemical composition. We find certain actions 'rewarding' because our brain gets an extra shot of the chemical hormone dopamine, a neurotransmitter that plays a big part in pleasure, reward and motivation.

Our dopamine circuits in particular are the brain's way of getting us to do things important for survival. Sex, which I'd say is pretty necessary for reproducing our species, comes with a huge burst of neurochemical reward. So does eating, as does drinking alcohol and taking drugs. In all these cases, dopamine is released into the pleasure circuits in the brain.

Of course, like just about everything in life, it's not that simple. Our brains also reward us for higher purposes – including doing positive things for ourself and for others. As neuroscientist David J. Linden explains in *The Compass of Pleasure*, the neurochemistry of gratification is extremely complex. You get rewarded with a sensation of pleasure when you inject yourself with drugs, but you also feel a sense of reward when you act virtuously and say no to drugs. Go figure! Brain-imaging studies show that 'providing for a public good' – giving to charity, for example – activates 'the same neural pleasure circuit that's engaged by heroin or orgasm or fatty foods'.[1]

Make that change

So, the positive news is that we have some built-in chemical mechanisms that reward us for doing things that are good for us and for the people around us. As our Reboot Medical Advisory Board Member (and success story) Dr Carrie Diulus says, 'When you choose not to have a doughnut and instead to have something healthy and you feel good about that, you get a little bit of dopamine.' That's one reason she recommends keeping lists of things we do that are healthy. Keeping a diary or checklist of food or exercise, for example, gives you a feeling of satisfaction when you mark off your progress. It also shows that, unlike old dogs, we actually can learn new tricks.

Even though we have the neural hardware to learn new ones, however, old habits are still hard to break. They are literally patterns laid down in our networks of brain cells, like rivulets in the sand after a rainstorm.

Want a good exercise to see how habits affect every aspect of your life? Try sitting comfortably in a chair and crossing your arms. Stay there for a while until you feel relaxed and at ease. Then change your arms by crossing them the other way. Does that feel as comfortable? Probably not. You crossed your arms the first way because it's your habit and felt the most comfortable. The other way just doesn't feel right.

So how long does it take to change a habit? In the case of crossed arms, a couple of weeks of crossing them the other way every time you sit down. For the bigger things, such as changing your habits of eating or exercising, or kicking an addiction, it's probably going to take more time. How long? As long as it takes for you to feel comfortable with your new routine. For some people that means a few weeks, for others a few months – and for others a few years. We are all different, but for all of us it's possible to change.

The important thing to be aware of is how powerful old habits are. When you start to change your food habits and you get that initial burst of energy and well-being from juicing and eating plants, you might think you've got it licked. But as you get further away from your Reboot and that initial surge of progress, and you come under the stress of living, it's not uncommon to slip back to your old ways. It's like you're a record needle: a big enough push and you skip back to an old groove.

If you want to sustain your health, your job is to keep the needle in its new groove and not let it jump backwards – and to move it back into place when it does.

Some useful techniques

When you come right down to it, eating is just a behaviour. What you're learning about in terms of good nutrition and healthy living is wonderful, but in the end it comes down to how you act. Change your behaviour and you change your food habits.

One of the key insights from a series of studies by Duke University psychologist David Neal and his colleagues is that once habits are established, they have little to do with our goals or motivations in life. They believe that everyday habits are far more likely to be changed by changing the 'triggers' of those largely unconscious behaviours – things such as time of day and location – than by knowledge or will-power.[2]

A lot of people, in fact, think it takes enormous will-power to succeed at breaking bad habits and replacing them with a sustainable healthy lifestyle. Certainly a little bit of discipline helps, but it's not all about will-power. It's just as much about being smart as it is about being tough, and the smarter you are, the less tough you have to be. The trick is to tilt the system in your favour. Here are some suggestions.

1 Slow it down.

One way to change your eating habits is literally to slow down. It takes about 20 minutes for your body to respond to the clues of satiation, and to reach the state of satiety or feeling full and no longer hungry. So if you eat fast, you generally pack in more food than you need – and certainly more than if you take your time and start to feel full before that huge serving in front of you is polished off.

There are different ways to slow things down. If you treat your food with a bit more reverence – something we talked about in changing your relationship with food – that slows things down. You might want to take more time chewing your food, which research shows makes digestion easier and helps your intestines absorb more nutrients. It's also another way to savour your meal a bit more.

In *Fat, Sick & Nearly Dead 2*, I talked with Cornell food researcher Professor Brian Wansink about some of the discoveries he writes about in his book *Mindless Eating*. One of the experiments that made headlines a couple of years ago took place in a branch of Hardee's fast food chain. Wansink and a colleague dimmed the lights and played mellow jazz in one section of the restaurant. Compared to the patrons in the noisy, bright areas of the restaurant, the special-section diners ate more slowly. And even though they ended up spending more time at the table, they ate less food – about 18 per cent less. Same food, same order, just a slower pace.[3]

You can apply this lesson to your home. Turn down the lights a little bit, or turn off that TV blaring in the background. Don't do anything but eat while you're eating, and consciously slow it all down.

2 Break the pattern.

Another insight that Duke psychologist Neal came up with is that deliberately changing your patterns of normal behaviour can help break habits. In one study, movie-goers only stopped eating a bucket of stale popcorn they were given when asked to use their 'non-dominant' hand – left instead of right for most of us. Neal calls this interrupting 'the pattern and context' of a habit. It can apply to your night-time snacking habits, for example. Just by changing where you sit to watch TV, or wherever you normally sit when having a snack, can increase your chances of successfully breaking a habit. What you've got to do, says Neal, is 'disrupt' the patterns that reinforce mindless habits, which are largely unconscious actions. Once you break the pattern, you've got a much better chance to bring your behaviour under 'intentional control'.[4]

3 Change the size.

Changing your immediate environment is much easier than changing your habits by using will-power. No one knows this better than Professor Wansink, who spent decades researching why we eat so much without thinking about it. He reckons most of us gain weight over the years because we mindlessly consume about 10 per cent too many calories every day. Catch these bad habits and you'll lose weight instead.

Wansink found that a lot of eating has to do with external signals and cues, not what our bodies – or even our conscious minds – tell us. Take serving size. Wansink observed that Americans are generally heavier than Europeans. Why? One simple reason: Americans tend to serve larger portions at meals than Europeans, both at home and in restaurants. Then they tend to clean their plates, taking the cues of satiation not from their stomachs but from their eyes, regardless of how much is served. Serve more, they eat more. So, just by serving a little less . . . you get the idea.

Granted, this seems sort of obvious. More subtle is the effect of container size on your brain. Large containers make it look like there's less food, and small containers make it look like there's more food. And that's how people experience it. If you give someone a large bucket of popcorn before the movie, they will eat more than if you give them a small or medium-sized bucket. If you give them a large glass, they will drink more. If you give them large plates, they will eat more. Every time.

This size factor also works when it comes to boxes. For example, if you buy the largest box of cereal, you'll eat more than if you're pouring from the smaller box. The same goes for ice cream; serve yourself from a regular-sized container and you'll eat less than if you're digging into a large tub. So spoon your servings into a bowl; you'll eat less than if you eat straight from the container. And try finding plates that are slightly smaller. It's a subtle difference that will make a big impact over time.

4 Keep it out of sight.

Remember the punchline to the old joke about the seafood diet? 'If I see food, then I eat it.' The sight of food is a powerful stimulus, something that advertisers know all too well. For some people the sight of food actually stimulates the pancreas into releasing insulin, preparing for a blast of sugar. That insulin release lowers the blood sugar level and makes you feel hungrier.

So one big way to change your eating habits is just to keep things out of sight. Sounds simple, but it works. In one case Wansink tracked office assistants who were given a jar of Hershey's Kisses as a gift for Secretary's Week. If the jar sat in front of them on their desks, they ate more than if the jar was on a filing cabinet across the room. If the jar was actually hidden, let's say inside a filing cabinet drawer, they ate fewer still.[5]

You can take this to the extreme, of course, perhaps by not walking down the street where your favourite bakery sits, or not driving past your local McDonald's. That may sound a little impractical, but at the very least you should reverse-engineer your kitchen and home so that everything tempting is out of sight. Studies show that the first things you see when you open the cupboard are three to five times more likely to be consumed than those you don't immediately see.

5 Make it hard to get.

Part of what was being measured in the secretary experiment was the convenience factor. If you have to walk across the room to get chocolate, you're going to eat less than if it's sitting on your desk. The more convenient the food, the more likely we are to consume it.

Our nutritionist Stacy Kennedy likes to cite a study where men were given the choice of taking two pills a day or eating two apples a day to counteract prostate cancer. Even if they were told the apples were equally or more effective, they always chose the pills. As she says, 'We have reached the point where convenience has a seat at the table in this culture more than it has in any other culture.'

This seems so obvious, doesn't it? But when it comes to overeating, knowing that reducing convenience can also reduce consumption is something we should use to our advantage. Why make your relationship with food one of struggle, of you versus temptation? If you have a packet of Oreos in your cupboard and it's right in your face when you open the door, it sets up a kind of contest of will-power. If you have to go to the shops to buy the Oreos, you're far less likely to eat them – especially since most cravings are gone in about 20 minutes.

6 One step at a time.

It's hard enough changing any particular habit, for me or anybody else. So it makes sense that it's even harder to wake up one morning and say that you're going to change everything, starting today. I think it's easier to change in small ways at first and build new habits one step at a time.

One of the ways to set yourself up for a relapse into old ways is to take on too much at once. It's a big reason most diets fail. You set up this entirely new regime of eating, one that's often uncomfortable if not downright unpleasant, and then you cling to it for dear life while you're losing weight. Once you've lost your weight, you go right back to the way you ate previously . . . heck, you can't wait to get back there.

One of the reasons I think that a Reboot is so effective is that it changes your relationship with food in a short period of time. Finish a Reboot that lasts 15 days or longer and I guarantee you will have a new-found love of fruits and veggies. (I can make the assumption that you didn't particularly care for them prior to your Reboot or you wouldn't be Rebooting.) Nonetheless, if your old habits around food still exist, you'll slowly find yourself eating fewer and fewer plants after the Reboot, and then you'll be looking at another failed diet. The diet didn't fail you; it was the after-the-diet diet that failed you.

So here's the thing: you don't even have to Reboot. You can start by eating more fruits and vegetables. You can change your habits around food more gradually and you will still get healthy and lose weight. It won't be nearly as fast as on a Reboot, but if you make lasting changes, you will make lasting health gains and weight losses.

7 The good stuff first.

A lot of us eat like we're kids. I certainly did. You know – where you push the vegetables out of the way and eat the meat first? A good way to change your eating habits is to reverse that order.

I recommend drinking a full glass of water before each meal; this way you won't confuse hunger with thirst, and you won't feel as empty. Then, when it comes to the other stuff on the plate, just eat the greens and/or salad first. Maybe you'll feel a little fuller by the time you get to the meat or the pasta.

You can also try replacing foods that are not nutritious by adding healthier ones. One of the vendors we work with at Reboot with Joe was inspired to replace his afternoon snack with a green juice. Just by having that juice instead of a piece of cake or a chocolate bar when his energy was flagging, he lost weight and had more energy in the afternoon. Just like when you identify your trigger foods and your treat foods, focus on amplifying what's going well in your diet. There might be a lot of things we're doing well, so let's not declare the whole thing a bloody disaster.

8 Start fresh.

You can get positive momentum going in a single day, and I think the best time to start is first thing in the morning. I try to approach each new day as if I'm waking up from a mini famine. I want to put in my system only the best, which means as much plant food as possible. Every now and then I go with an omelette because I think it's OK to have a little animal protein once in a while, but I try to focus on plants for the first part of the day – juice, fruit, oatmeal or maybe a smoothie.

Now, I'm fairly certain that if I'd got up and eaten a whole packet of Oreos for breakfast, I would have found it really hard to go and eat something healthy after that. You kind of feel like eating crap all day rather than your veggies. In the same way that you can teach your taste buds to prefer veggies, you can also unteach them, and pretty fast. And it triggers a pattern with me that I've started poorly, that I've let myself down, that it's all over, that I might as well crash.

Whatever that syndrome is – whether I'm trying to keep that manufactured bliss point going, or I'm low on energy, or I just don't like myself – I find that if I start my day by consuming more plants, I'm able to balance myself out and cruise better throughout the whole day. It certainly leaves me less prone to sugar crashes, where I feel like I need a piece of chocolate or some kind of sugar hit to pick me up.

9 Build the momentum.

If you start the day with a glass of juice and maybe some exercise, that goes a long way toward giving you the momentum to face the rest of the day's challenges in a healthy way. It puts the wind at your back. The same goes for small victories and constructive changes. They reinforce each other and you start a positive spiral. If you take the one-step-at-a-time approach, of changing things incrementally at first – pruning the bushes, so to speak – you begin to change the momentum. A whole lot of little moments can make a great moment. The star player in a football match doesn't get that accolade for just one moment; it's about a lot of moments. It's the momentum of the little moments.

Building positive momentum, in a single day or over many days, is a powerful lever for changing food habits. You create a positive spiral of self-reinforcing actions that are good for you. It creates a kind of pride. If you go to the gym, or for a walk in the woods, or for a hike in the hills, or to play tennis – whatever – when you drive home you'll find you're more likely to make that extra effort to drive to the smoothie bar. Or you'll make that effort to head to the vegan restaurant. Whereas if you're not in the positive spiral and you see a burger bar, well, bugger hell, you'll go in there.

10 Beware the influencers.

In the process of changing your food habits, it's important to understand the psychology of external cues that influence what and how much we eat. We've discussed these in terms of the inducements of advertisers, and in terms of serving and container size, but not in terms of the social standards that condition our habits.

I don't know about you, but I'll never stop hearing my parents' voices telling me to finish everything on my plate because the people in Africa are starving. My mum would actually say, 'You are now part of the clean plate club.' It was a job, and I felt rewarded. So do most of us in the West today: studies show that on average we eat 92 per cent of what we put on our plates. In some cultures a clean plate is considered an insult to the host or hostess, since it implies that you didn't get enough. Not in our world.

Obese people, it turns out, are more sensitive to external cues and influencers than non-obese people. In his work studying the eating habits of the overweight, the late psychologist Stanley Schachter did one experiment showing how obese subjects kept in a windowless room ate more when the wall clocks were speeded up. They were influenced more by the external cues of the 'time for dinner' than by their own feelings of hunger. If the clock said it was time to eat, so be it.[6]

So you need to stop playing by the rules of others. Don't eat to be polite, or just because someone is making the offer, or because it's dinnertime. Start to be more of a maverick when it comes to socially accepted food habits. And listen to your body instead of the clock.

11 Keep a list.

There is some part of me that doesn't like keeping lists. It seems a little too controlling. But doctors and fitness instructors know how powerful keeping a list can be for sticking to an exercise or eating programme.

There are two ways you can go. The first is the elimination list, where you write down all the things you want to get done, then cross them off as you go. It's a great way to get organized and a great way to visualize what you want to accomplish. For that matter, it's also a de-stresser, because once you write down what you need to do, you don't have to think about it as much, or worry about forgetting something important. The satisfaction comes with crossing off each successive item.

The other way is to keep a record of things as you get them done. This is particularly effective for exercise regimes and athletic training because of the tremendous reinforcement you get recording your progress. It gives you a sense of fulfilment and self-esteem as you see your number of reps increase, or the length of your running time expand. It also keeps you honest and reminds you to keep to your routine.

The same goes for food and keeping a food diary. It makes you think about each thing you eat, since you're going to be writing it down, and it lets you see honestly how much you're really cramming in. In this way, keeping a list is a great way to guard against mindless eating. If you're keeping a record of your weight and how you feel, you can also see the relationship between food and your weight and health.

You can keep your own notebook or diary, or use one of the many online apps, or even wear a fitness device, such as the Jawbone UP or FitBit wristbands. We have both a tracker and an app for tracking your Reboot and how you're eating after your Reboot (visit www.rebootwithjoe.com).

Everything is relative

As you change your food habits, your perception of taste starts to shift. Once you get off the sugar train, you begin to experience flavours that were too subtle to notice before. Without sugar to make your taste buds jaded, fruits become sweeter to the taste.

What you are experiencing is a shifting baseline of what we consider sweet or salty. Once you have recalibrated your sense of taste, there is a balance and a limit where too much of a treat actually doesn't taste very good; it can taste sickeningly sweet or bitterly salty.

We adjust to the world like this all the time. A good example of how relative our perceptions are is a place called Kents Cavern, a large cave in southwest England. Now a tourist attraction, the cavern was occupied by primitive humans for thousands of years. What they liked was its constant year-round temperature of 14°C (58°F). In the winter, when the outside temperature dropped below freezing, it felt warm inside, and vice versa in the summer.

I experienced this concept of relativity quite dramatically when I was a teenager. I was 19 when I attended a concert by Spandau Ballet in the Sydney Entertainment Centre. We were sitting way in the back, and behind us was a group of girls my age. One girl was dancing so much that her glasses flew off. They fell onto my chair and I put them on as a joke. All of a sudden I could see the stage, and that purple blur became a drum set and a guitarist and a dancer. It had never occurred to me that I needed glasses. All of a sudden I was awake to the fact that my eyesight wasn't perfect. I thought everyone saw the way I did. Needless to say, I've worn glasses from that day forward.

The point is that sometimes you don't realize what you don't know. Having a large pizza every night and feeling a certain way can seem normal if you don't know what it's like to feel healthy and strong and good. And if you don't know what it's like to feel healthy and strong and good, you don't know that it's the pizza that's been holding you back.

This is why a Reboot is so effective in helping to achieve new food habits – it creates a new benchmark for your experience of eating. During a juice Reboot, your body starts to change its sensibilities towards nutritious foods, and starts to enjoy and even yearn for the nutritious foods that help your cells to function the way they should. Your sense of taste gets recalibrated. Afterwards, nutritious foods not only make you feel better, they start tasting better to you. These are actual changes in your brain chemistry, in the same way that runners experience a 'high' from their exercise, and symptoms of withdrawal when they skip their exercise routines. Once you get used to a better diet, you'll miss it when it you stop. But only for a while. It's still up to you to make those new habits just that.

HOW TO BREAK FOOD HABITS

Ready to identify and break your food habits? Try the following:

1 **Change your dinner environment.** Try turning down the volume at dinnertime. Instead of eating around a blaring TV set, eat at the table to some quiet music. And slow down the pace. Chew more. Savour your food.

2 **Change your dinner plates.** It may seem like a small thing, but Professor Wansink found that smaller plates meant smaller meals with the same level of satisfaction. So try using smaller plates, and serve yourself a little bit less than normal. Just 10 per cent less will make a big difference over time.

3 **Change your kitchen environment.** If there are problem foods for you, just don't stock them at home. Or keep them out of sight. Don't make changing your food habits a contest of will.

4 **Change your mealtime patterns.** Start by drinking water and eating your greens first, not last. This will fill you up a bit and slow you down a little with the foods you know are going to add on useless calories.

5 **Change your breakfast.** Start your first meal of the day with a big glass of green juice. Go ahead with your normal breakfast – or what you want of it – after that. But start the day with a good, healthy feeling.

6 **Keep a food diary.** One of the best ways to understand how different foods affect you, and what sort of long-term eating habits work best for you, is to keep a record of literally everything you eat. This helps to make mindless eating habits conscious ones too.

It has not always been easy or smooth for Mike Kyles-Villalobos, but since he began his first Reboot more than two years ago, he always returns to what he calls 'the balance'. And that has allowed him to maintain a healthy lifestyle, and sustain his weight loss of more than 7½ stone (110 pounds).

'I don't want to say that it's perfect every day, but I am consistently trying to eat healthy and incorporate healthier foods,' says Mike, who works as a school therapist. 'I keep harkening back to *Fat, Sick & Nearly Dead*, where Joe asked if he'd be able to achieve and maintain a balance.'

One thing Mike has done is to use substitutes for his former comfort foods, such as chicken salad instead of a hamburger, or bean chips instead of French fries. 'I go the healthier-version route. It's almost like watching the sanitised version of an X-rated movie. The X-rated version is like fried chicken, mashed potatoes – all that stuff. Eating healthy is like watching the clean version of the movie. You still get to see it.'

Mike, who is a self-confessed food addict, says that two things help bring him back when he falls into what he calls 'the dark, deep hole' of binge-eating: friends and inspiration.

'When I started my big Reboot [which lasted 70 days] my friends and family thought I was crazy. In the beginning it was like, "Is that even healthy?" But when they saw my weight coming off, and saw me being passionate about what I was doing, it was nothing but support. Whenever I was about to break, it was like, "Mike, keep it going, stick to your goal!"'

Now Mike incorporates his circle of friends into his new lifestyle. Before his Reboot he avoided exercise. Now he goes to the gym several days a week, and on frequent hikes into the hills near his home – along with friends.

'Eating healthy is very much a lifestyle, and one where

you can slip and fall very easily,' he says. 'You have to have like-minded people around you. You can't hang around people who eat junk food all day. That's going to send you right back down into the hole. A lot of my friends, the people I hang around with now, eat healthy. They want to live better, happier lives . . . I believe that who we surround ourselves with is who we become.'

Having said that, Mike says it's unrealistic to think you're going to eat something nutritious all the time. 'Not every day am I doing a strictly plant based diet . . . When you're hanging out with friends at happy hour, you're not going to order a salad. You're going to grub out. It's knowing when you're able to say no, and training yourself. It's a mind game.'

That's where inspiration comes in.

'I have a shirt that I fit into when I'm 220–230 pounds [15½ stone – he was 24½ stone (345 pounds) when he Rebooted]. I know I can fit into this shirt. So when I go down that deep, dark hole for four or five or six days, I see if I can fit into that shirt. If I can't, I say, "Mike you're going right back to where you were. Let's go back and Reboot." That's how I keep myself in shape. At one point I had to go up a size in my pants because I wasn't eating right, and that was after a week and a half of eating crazy. So I had to get out the *Fat, Sick & Nearly Dead* DVD, make my juice and commit myself.'

Mike also makes inspirational playlists, one song for each day he plans to spend on his Reboot. 'I thank God that Joe called it a Reboot because it makes sense. You're not dieting, you are just retraining your body, bringing it back to the factory settings. It's also retraining your mind.'

That's important because Mike wrestles with the voice inside his head, the one that chimes in when he eats poorly and tells him, 'Well, you've already messed up now, so you might as well go into it deeper.' Mike thinks that voice comes from how people are raised in America – to be competitive with others, right from the earliest experiences on sports teams. 'Once that competitive spirit gets inside ourselves and we fail, we immediately revert back to how we felt as little kids, like, "Oh, I didn't do as good as Johnny, I didn't get first place," so you beat yourself up as just worthless.'

This sense of winners and losers is everywhere, he says, including in our TV programming. 'It's like reality TV,' says Mike. 'Everything is a competition. When you're not the best, you go home. The winner has this cocky spirit about them, but you never see the story of the person who failed . . . Nobody cares about the losers, so why would anyone care about me if I mess up? So we go ahead and crash.'

In the end, says Mike, the only competition worth winning is the one with yourself, to achieve a sense of satisfaction. 'You want the feeling of having accomplished this, that you beat the demon inside your head . . . Once you tame that beast inside your mind, then you have everything conquered.'

4

EMBRACE COMMUNITY (Get a Little Help From Your Friends)

I spend a lot of my life these days on the road, living in hotel rooms, travelling to cities where people want to learn more about Rebooting and what it takes to live a healthier life. What amazes me the most are the number of people who reach out with stories about their successes with juicing and plant-based diets. I never get tired of hearing these, and I am always deeply touched.

What I've learned the most from these wonderful, inspiring people is that when it comes to your last two feet of freedom – the decision of what to put in your mouth – the right choice is a whole lot easier to make when you are not alone. When you have support. When you are connected.

I've learned this literally out on the streets, when I've talked with successful Rebooters, because I really try to drill down to the core of why they've done well. And, except in very rare cases, they all have a support network – 99.9 per cent. When they don't, they start to fail, just as Phil Staples did. Phil, the truck driver in *Fat, Sick & Nearly Dead*, successfully maintained his 18-stone (250-pound) weight loss and health improvements until his divorce and loneliness sent him on a downward spiral.

Phil is far from unique, by the way. Globally, the number of one-person households has risen by nearly a third over the last decade. Some countries are lonelier than others, but the Western nations are all pretty comparable. As of 2012, one-person households accounted for 25 per cent of the Australian total,[1] 27 per cent in the USA,[2] 28 per cent in Canada,[3] and 29 per cent in the UK.[4]

The reasons for this vary. People are marrying later in life, and not getting remarried as quickly after a divorce. Older married people who survive their spouses aren't moving back in with their children. Our mass migration from traditional rural communities to modern industrial cities has had a lot to do with it. And the social security provided by modern welfare states has enabled more people to live alone.

The result is a world rife with loneliness, where social networks that were part of how we lived for thousands of years have all but disappeared. As our friend and author Dr Dean Ornish says, 'People used to get that [social connectivity] from their extended families or their neighbourhoods, with two or three generations of people [living together], or a church or synagogue that they would go to regularly, or a sense of safety at work, with a job you've been at for many years. Many people don't have any of those things because there's been such a radical disruption of these social networks . . . the real primal need is for connection and community.'

The need for community is so basic that without it we simply get sick. It doesn't seem to matter whether we get our sense of community from belonging to a group of friends or from intimacy with a significant other, but we need it. Some health pundits separate intimacy – the love you share for someone very close – from community. I don't see them so much as separate as different steps along the continuum of connectedness. It's like with family. Most people have at least the connection of the nuclear family – a mother or father, a sister or brother, a son or daughter – and that can be as beneficial as being part of a larger community.

Either way, what the research says is this: people who are lonely are three to ten times as likely to get sick and die prematurely as those who are part of a community of relatives and friends. One study showed that people who didn't have family or friends were much less likely to engage in physical activity. This made them less active, less mobile and even lonelier, in a self-reinforcing negative spin of deteriorating health.

The opposite spin is also true. As Dr Ornish notes, 'People are much more likely to make and maintain lifestyle choices that are life-enhancing than ones that are self-destructive when they feel that sense of community.' Another groundbreaking study showed that low-quality relationships with friends and family were as bad for health as smoking 15 cigarettes a day or drinking heavily. In fact, they were even worse than a lack of exercise or obesity!

The power of the group

In the practical world of making good choices to sustain your health, the breakdown of social networks – scattered families, lack of friends – makes it much, much harder to succeed. You just can't do it alone. Well, maybe you can, but good luck trying. Although we may enter and leave this world alone, while we're here, we're flying anything but solo.

One of the things we've found at Reboot is that having like-minded folks in your circle, people who can offer you understanding and support, is critical when it comes to making the changes you need to make. We call this circle of support, be it one person or a dozen, your community. It comprises family, friends and the social groups you join. If you don't have this community, you feel pretty much alone and isolated in your struggle. But knowing that someone understands what you're going through makes it much easier to bear.

This is not a unique insight. It's been 80 years now since the founding of the most famous group therapy organization, Alcoholics Anonymous (AA). The idea was to help people addicted to alcohol to come to terms with their addiction and its effect on themselves and their loved ones, by working through it with help from others who'd gone through the experience. And it's been very effective.

What AA meetings pioneered was the power of community support, working in a safe, caring space provided by groups of people who have undergone what you're going through. In these environments you know you're not on your own; rather, you are surrounded by folks who empathize.

For some people, realizing they are not alone – becoming aware that there are many, many people going through the same thoughts and feelings – is a life-changing experience. We tend to think that everyone else is having a great time in life and that we're the only ones walking around tripping on our bottom lips, feeling sorry for ourselves. When we see that's not the case, it's like a huge burden is lifted.

'I'm new to the site and felt I needed to be surrounded with people on the same mission as myself,' is what one Rebooter posted on our website. 'It is good to read that someone else has also begun the same way as me and that I am not alone. Thank you,' posted another. And still another, 'Good for you for starting, and no matter how you do it, you're working at making a better and healthier you. Never feel that you're alone. It's so easy to feel like a failure, isn't it? Just last night I was telling my husband that no one ever has to beat me up or kick me when I'm down . . . because I do that to myself . . .'

We need connectivity in this world of seven billion people. When it comes to making a positive change for yourself or sustaining one you've already made, feeling alone or isolated is a downward drag. The quickest path to self-destruction is to feel that no one cares about you or understands your struggle. How many times have you thought, 'If no one else gives a damn, why should I?' Finding and joining a group of fellow travellers takes you in the opposite direction, on the road to health.

Outside yourself

There are lots of other potent forces at work when you join a community, beyond the wonderful feeling that others understand and care about you. One of them is what happens when you talk about things out loud, and make promises not just to yourself but also to others around you.

When we were making the film *Fat, Sick & Nearly Dead*, I came to realize this. I'd never made a film before and didn't know how to act, so when I looked down that lens, I would imagine I was talking to a family somewhere in the Midwest, or to a couple in Perth, or to an individual sitting at home in Canada – to a community out there that was watching. And the more I thought this way, the more I understood that I had to succeed for them.

At the time I didn't fully perceive how important this was. But after the film was released, and I was on the road promoting it, I realized that this was my community, my support group, and the people I could not let down. It was all the individuals who came up and shared their stories: a woman who no longer suffered from diabetes; a man who no longer had Crohn's disease; a mother who had lost 14 stone (200 pounds) and could now play with her grandchildren. People who thanked me for literally saving their lives. One was a soldier who had lost both legs while serving in Afghanistan. I almost cried when he thanked me for the difference that Rebooting made in his life. It was a humbling experience for me. When you hear people like this, who tell you that you've inspired them to change their lives, how can you possibly give up? They inspire me.

I think there are really two levels of communication we must manage in our lives: the internal communication and the external communication. The internal is the voice inside, how we talk to ourselves; the external is the voice we use to talk to other people.

Like being asleep and being awake, I don't think we can have one without the other. We can have all sorts of conversations with ourselves about exercise and diet and how best to act, but talking about these things with others makes it like a pledge to them. I know when I tell someone that I'm going to go for a run tomorrow, I'm more likely to do it, especially if they are around to see whether I did. Or, better yet, if I make a date to go on a walk or hike with someone, I'm way more likely to follow through with the exercise. You can image how powerful that is when you've made a promise to millions of viewers.

So part of the magic that community brings is the power of making a commitment to someone – or some group – beyond ourselves. Fooling ourselves is one of the easiest things in the world to do. It's something we do every day, on an almost hourly basis. It's much harder to fool other people, especially after you've put it out there, so to speak. Telling yourself you're going to make a change is one thing: you can talk yourself out of that. But making a pledge to a group is very different: now you're letting other people down. As humans, we hate to do that.

One of the more successful if unusual self-help groups for weight loss is called the Trevose Behavior Modification Program. It was launched in 1970 by a formerly obese insurance executive and named after the Philadelphia suburb where members attended weekly group sessions. It continues today in and around Philly.

It was (and is) a very strict programme, where you announce weight-loss goals and stick to them, no excuses. The commitment to others is so intense that if you fail to meet your publicly declared goals, you are kicked out of the group. Pretty rough stuff. In a study they did in the 1990s, less than half the participants made it to the two-year mark. But guess what? Those who hung in lost an average of 19 per cent of their body weight in those two years, and pretty much kept it off (17 per cent) after five years if they were still on board.[5]

We're a little gentler and less judgemental at Reboot, but the message is fundamentally the same: if you say you're going to do something out loud to your community – be it friends, family or a self-help group – you're more likely to stick to it than if you say it just to yourself. Somehow the external communication makes it real.

When you think about it, that approach applies pretty

much to anything you think or say. The conversations we have with ourselves are not reality, whereas conversations we have with others are. How many times have you thought about something that you'd like to yell out in a public place, or at an event, or a meeting, or in a social group? Fortunately for me, that internal communication is not reality. If I shouted out half the things I've thought of, wondering what would happen, people would think I was bonkers and should be locked up. Saying things – and that includes texting, tweeting, Facebooking, etc. – tends to make them real, which is another reason to embrace community.

Lessons from our elders

So just how important is a sense of community for a long and healthy life?

In his book *The Blue Zones, National Geographic* writer Dan Buettner looks at five communities around the world where the people remain healthy and vibrant into their old age – and where an astonishingly high number of the people live to be 100 years old or more.

While diets may vary (though all are plant-based), and habits may vary (some sleep late and others rise early), the one absolute constant is community. All of these healthy, long-lived people have a strong network of family and friends with whom they interact regularly, and upon whom they can rely. It's what the centenarians on the Japanese island of Okinawa call their *moai* – their group of lifelong friends.[6] Contrast that with the UK, where the average Briton has only three true friends.[7] In America it's even worse, where the average person has only two close friends.[8]

Besides the stress-busting security of the emotional and even financial safety net that a *moai* supplies, these close-knit social groups provide another important function – a sense of purpose or place. It's what the Okinawans call *ikigai*, or their role in the community. It's the reason why they get up each morning. The absence of *ikigai* is a big reason why mortality rates soar for people who retire – they no longer have a sense of purpose.[9]

In the early 1990s I attended the wedding of one of my best mates, an Australian who married a beautiful woman from Thailand. The ceremony took place in Nan, her village way up in the north, close to the Golden Triangle. When I arrived I couldn't believe the remoteness of the place. It was like going back 500 years in time. I remember seeing all these children who spent hours each morning trudging down to a well and hauling water back in buckets and pails – all the water needed by the entire village each day.

Now, as Mr Joe Cross, the man from Sydney in the modern world, I had the solution. I figured it couldn't cost more than a few thousand dollars to install a pump and some pipe tubing. That would get the water up the hill to the village and solve the problem.

I was doing well financially at the time, so I went to the village boss, a woman, and offered my solution as a gift. Do you know what she said? 'Thanks for the kind offer,' she told me, 'but the village respectfully declines. If we accept this gift, what will the children do?' You see, this lugging of the water was their job, their role, what their older brothers and sisters and parents had done before them. It was what integrated them into the community and made them a valuable part of it. Thanks, but no thanks.

This got me wondering about the breakdown of modern

community. Is it down to the fact that we all need a role to play? When we don't have a role, we feel a little bit alone; we feel rudderless, and we look for ways to fill that gap. Think of how many snack-food advertisements show people having fun together. Do we reach for the processed food in the hope it can fill that lonely gap? I know that's what Phil Staples did when he returned to eating fast food.

In the movie *Fat, Sick & Nearly Dead 2*, I spend some time visiting an exceptional high school in Brooklyn, New York City. The school – now called the High School for Public Service – was previously a sinkhole of violence and terrible drop-out rates. Among other initiatives, one thing the principal did was to create a community garden that the students would plant, sustain and harvest. Participation in the garden gave the students a hands-on sense of purpose and contribution. Using this and other mechanisms to foster a sense of community, the principal reversed the school's decline and made it top-ranking.

When I grew up in Sydney, I was raised as a Catholic and I attended St Ignatius College in Riverview. Our school was run by the Jesuits. St Ignatius of Loyola, the father of the order, had been a soldier in the early 1500s until a cannon-ball shattered his legs. During his long months of recuperation, he read about the life of Jesus and the saints, and decided to become a soldier of God instead of a soldier of war.

I mention this because of what the order espoused, which was the idea that we are here to serve others. Their motto translates literally as 'Men for Others' (they weren't too keen on including women in those days), and it meant that we are here to be of service. It's the same philosophy that was taught by Mahatma Gandhi. In helping others you find yourself.

Community works that way as well. It's not just a matter

of what you take from the group; it's also what you give. When it comes to reaching out and joining your local community, working as a volunteer can be just as beneficial as joining up to look for help and support. Coming from a social species as we do, we all feel an innate need to contribute to the group. It's part of what makes us human and what defines us as a species.

Finding your wingman

'Family values' is one of the most overused expressions today, especially by politicians in the USA. But the appeal of that nostalgic trigger, and why elected officials use it so often, is because in the not-too-distant past families stayed together. And not just families, but whole communities. In small towns and villages everybody knew each other. There were extended families of both relatives and friends. The sense of community was palpable, and that close-knit world was healthy for us.

Why these community networks broke apart in the modern world has a great deal to do with the mass migration of people from rural communities to urban centres. You can see it going on right now in China, where people from village communities are leaving in droves and heading for the huge cities. It's a speeded-up version of what happened in the West over the last 200 or 300 years: people moving far from home to find a better, more prosperous way of life. What has broken down our social networks is the promise (also usually broken) of a future that's going to be a better place if it has running water and power, appliances and a supermarket with many thousands of items on the shelves.

The result is a world where families no longer stay together, where children move far away from their parents once they grow up, and where all our childhood friends scatter to the wind. This has become the norm, not the exception, and I admit it sounds pretty bad.

But there's a silver lining to this. I think there is a trade-off between the old ways of small towns with extended families, and the modern way of nuclear families and a lot more solo households. The very technology that split up the old communities gives us the power to join or create new ones. The silver lining is that we now have a choice. It's like the old expression that you can choose your friends but not your family. In the past you couldn't choose your community; it was the place where you grew up. When you escaped to the big city, you could.

Look at it this way. You've got maybe six or seven big lifestyle choices that contribute to your health problems. They involve stress, smoking, alcohol, food, exercise and intimacy.

Each one of us has to look at those categories and ask, 'How is my community helping or hindering these things in my life?' If I don't want to drink, yet I hang out with people who just love to go to the pub and drink, maybe it's time to switch communities. If you let your friends know you're trying to get healthy, do they show up at the door with an ice cream or do they enthusiastically try your latest green juice recipe and suggest a walk?

Here's the thing. If you're part of a community that doesn't support a healthy lifestyle, that can be a problem. Studies show that our lifestyle choices are heavily influenced by the people we hang out with. One study of high school kids showed that if you are overweight but hang out with lean friends, you have a 60 per cent chance of losing weight within a year. If, on the other hand, you are borderline obese and hang out with obese friends, you have a 56 per cent chance of gaining weight during the year.[10]

The reasons we're susceptible to social influences aren't fully understood. There are a lot of chemical reactions going on that we don't understand yet. But the fact is that if you hang out with someone who is the most optimistic person you know, a super-happy person, you'll walk away feeling much better. And if you hang out with someone who supports what you're doing with your diet and your healthy lifestyle, you're going to find it much easier.

One thing that Russ Kennedy likes to say is that everyone needs a wingman. If you're lucky, this person is your significant other. But a lot of times this is not the case, so you've got to find that support person, especially at first. A friend who is going to go on the journey with you. Someone you can reach out to for advice. And someone who understands the programme – maybe someone experienced who can offer advice on how to tell your partner that the steak dinner he or she is planning to reward you with for 15 days of Rebooting isn't really a great reward.

A lot of people who start a Reboot get the 'Are you crazy?' reaction from people they're close to. Some even go on to say it can't be good for you, that it'll cause diabetes, that it will make your life miserable. A wingman is there to back you up instead of putting up roadblocks. A wingman is the person who supports you in moments of weakness.

Most people are familiar with having a wingman (or wingwoman) when it comes to exercise programmes. If you have a running partner who's watching out for you, they'll be the first to challenge you when you start to slacken. He or she is the person who says, 'Come on, don't be so lazy! Get off the couch, it's time for our run!' He or she is the one who says, as you speed-walk through the neighbourhood, 'No, let's not stop at that convenience store for a soda. Let's just keep going.'

When I was on the road promoting *Fat, Sick & Nearly Dead*, I really didn't have a wingman. Sometimes I felt terribly alone on the journey. But I eventually came to realize that my community – and my wingman – were all the people I came across; all those folks I couldn't let down were keeping an eye on me. It was like I had the eyes of big brothers and big sisters everywhere.

I remember one time about two years ago when I was in San Francisco. I had some free time, so I went by myself to see a movie, and decided to get some ice cream. You know I think that's OK when you're balanced, but this particular time I hadn't really earned it. Nonetheless, I went to the counter, ordered the ice cream and got myself a water. And when I went to pay, the guy who served me said, 'I didn't know Joe the Juicer ate ice cream.' That was all it took. I threw the ice cream in the bin. I said, 'Thanks, mate. You've helped me go instantly from wanting the ice cream to not wanting it.' That's what a wingman does – he or she helps you in your quest to sustain health, especially at the big crisis points.

Online solutions

Not everyone is as lucky as I was in finding a community of support. Some people have partners who actually want them to be unhealthy and dependent, or who simply like their lifestyle of food and drink. It's not common, but sometimes a Rebooter's marriage ends after a successful Reboot.

Hopefully, you won't have to go to such an extreme, but you might have to take a good hard look at your relationships. If your friends or loved ones can't provide the support you need to succeed, that's one thing; a lot of times these people come to support and even follow you once you've been successful. But if they actively undermine you, that's another matter. In that case, find a wingman, if not a larger community, who can be your partner in the efforts to find and sustain a healthy lifestyle.

Sometimes you have to look outside your immediate circle, especially in those early days of taking the tough, tentative steps toward a new, healthy lifestyle. One such place is online. Here's a great example of modern technology opening up pathways to new communities of like-minded people. Not only can online communities link you to people who can empathize, they can also make participants feel safe in a way that lets them be more honest than they might have been in person.

At www.rebootwithjoe.com we have an online community of nearly 300,000 members. Some of our members are Reboot veterans, others are just starting out on their journey to weight loss and health. You can find almost any kind of group in our community: Canuck Rebooters; Looking Good For Xmas; Fabulous Fatties; Saying Goodbye to 100 pounds or more; Juicing Our Way to Remission: Auto-immune Diseases; Juicing and Eating Disorders; Grieving Juicers; Veteran Juicers; even Gaming Geek Juicers. I could go on and on. The point is that we have someone else in our community who shares your interests, your issues and your concerns. And we at Reboot are continually in awe of the people in our community. They are incredibly caring, knowledgeable and, above all, inspiring.

The sharing of knowledge is another important reason to embrace community. It all goes back to the roots of who we are as human beings. In many ways we owe our success as a species to living and working together as a group – one reason why our brain rewards us for doing something that benefits the community. But we also succeeded as a group because we learned by seeing what others did. We could see the ones who were successful and the ones who weren't, and learn from the ones who were. It really did come down to one person who first ate the oyster; if that one brave (or stupid) person didn't die, then the rest could follow.

So we need community. We always have. We define ourselves in a social context, and we need to be intimately connected to other humans. Community is a vital ingredient for good physical and mental health, and without it we find that our sense of purpose and meaning is compromised. We become lonely and literally heartsick. When you become part of a community, what you'll discover is a sense of belonging, of self-worth and support, especially from those who share your goals and experience.

TIPS FOR GETTING MORE SUPPORT

Feel like you could use a little more community and support? Try the following:

1 **Volunteer!** Every town or city has groups that need volunteers. These may be churches, community kitchens, or even grassroots political organizations. Pick one that fits into your core interests and join up. You will find the old saying 'You get what you give' to be truer than you thought.

2 **Get regular exercise.** This is always beneficial to good health. It also provides an excuse to meet and mingle with others who are interested in good health. So try joining a gym and participating in some of the group classes. It's an excellent way to make like-minded friends who will keep you on your game.

3 **Join an evening class.** Adult evening classes are widely available in many different subjects. There are also postgraduate courses geared towards people with regular jobs. Remember your friends from schooldays? Schools and colleges are still great environments for bonding with people who have similar interests.

4 **Go online and join a like-minded community.** At www.rebootwithjoe.com there are numerous online communities you can join, where you will find sympathetic people who can help you through your tough times as you learn to live a healthier life. And you can help others too, which is its own reward.

YOU'VE GOT TO HAVE COMMUNITY
Bobby Brennan

Even before Bobby Brennan began his first juice fast, his community of family and friends were there to support him. About eight years ago, when he began approaching 35 stone (500 pounds), a close friend held what he called 'an intervention' to see what could be done to help. Since then, the support has only grown, going from weekly meetings at Weight Watchers to an online community of juicers that he says 'has made all the difference'.

Bobby, 41, is a professional musician who plays the bass. Unless he is on tour, playing with a band or in the orchestra pit for a Broadway play, he lives in Orlando, Florida. Eight years ago, when the dial showed an astonishing 494 pounds, he thought the scales he was on were broken.

That's when friend and fellow musician Michael Andrews gave him 'the talk', says Bobby. 'He just sat me down in the hotel room – we were out on tour at the time – and he said, "What are you doing? What's going on?" He didn't talk to me in a degrading way, like "Hey you're getting huge." He just said, "What's going on here? Let's correct this."'

Bobby knew his health was in danger. He was having a hard time carrying his bass, his back hurt, he was sweating like crazy, and he was constantly out of breath. So he joined Weight Watchers, which took him down to about 25 stone (350 pounds). That's when he 'plateaued' and couldn't seem to lose any more weight. And that's when his friend Michael also came across *Fat, Sick & Nearly Dead* and told him he should watch it.

'I was still working hard at losing weight, and doing this and that, but I'd gotten stuck. Then I got into juicing and that really changed a lot. That changed everything,' he says. Among other things, he learned about wholefoods and a plant-based diet. 'Before that it was, "Hey, this is 97 per cent fat-free, so it must be good." But it was a processed food, with processed sugar, and that's no good. Then I got into the juice.'

Among other things, Bobby immediately joined several online communities. 'I joined a couple of juice groups, a lot of them big fans of Joe. I joined because when you're doing this type of journey, we're all in it together. Sure, we're all on our own journey, but at the same time we all need to support one another.'

That was just the beginning of the help he got from friends, family and even co-workers. At the time he did his 60-day juice fast, Bobby was playing with the orchestra for a soon-to-be-Broadway production called *Enchanted*.

'We were doing a 12-week run; we had just started, and I was living with two cast members, two girls that were in the show,' he says. 'I explained that I was going to be juicing for the whole run. I told them, "Hey ladies, I'll try not to disturb you, but I'm going to be juicing. So just support me, and make sure I don't go off track. I want to stick to this." They said, "Twelve weeks? That's tough." But they were great. They just couldn't believe I was going to do it.'

Bobby did succeed, however – with a little encouragement from Joe Cross himself, who was doing a book tour nearby – and on the last day of the show got a big surprise.

'On the 100th show, which just happened to be my last day of juicing, the cast brought me out on stage. Instead of flowers they got me a big basket of kale and apples and vegetables. The audience didn't get it. It was like, "What are they giving him a bunch of vegetables for?" So I explained to the audience that I'd just finished 60 days of juicing. You could hear everyone in the crowd go, "Aaah..."'

Since then, Bobby has lost another 7 stone (100 pounds). He has joined a gym for daily workouts, become a regular at several juice bars, and has gone to the flipside of community support by becoming an adviser to newcomers. These include the instructors at his gym, tough guys who were amazed by his energy levels and who he can now bark at to 'suck it up'. He has also started his own blog, 'Fat Guy Drinks Juice', which has 600 followers.

'If you ask me what keeps me going now, it's people being inspired by me, people talking, people emailing me. I get emails from people all over, from India and from Germany. I can't fail these people . . . That's what's really motivating me to keep going strong – I'm setting an example for others, just as others set examples for me. That's really, really important. It's also really important to let people know what you're doing . . . You've got to have a community.'

5

MAINTAIN THE MACHINE
(Follow the Upkeep Manual)

Words cannot describe the magnificence and the magic that is the human body. Few things in the universe are as amazing. With hundreds of billions of specialized cells, the body is capable not only of great feats of intelligence and creativity, but also of repairing itself. Think about that: an organism that can restore itself when damaged. No machine we've ever created can do that.

Most of what we discuss in this book is about the energy and information we put into the organism we call our body. Let's call this blend of information and energy 'fuel'. And for the sake of explanation, let's call our body a 'machine'. Better fuel means better performance and a lot less damage along the way. But better fuel alone is not enough. You also have to maintain the machine, running it through its paces to keep everything working properly. Then you have to give it the right amount of downtime, so that internal repairs can take place.

What these functions come down to in human terms are exercise and sleep. In one sense, these two states of action and inaction are like the bookends to our lives, the two extremes. One bookend is all about being flat on your back, where you are supposed to be unconscious. The other is where your heartrate is 175 and you're running up a steep hill. Most of the time you're in the middle ground, sitting at your desk, or driving your car, or casually window-shopping as you walk down the street.

I put them together here because they're really two sides of the same coin, more closely related than you would think (the same part of the brain, the thalamus, actually controls both movement and sleep). If you don't get regular exercise, you're going to find it harder to get a good night's sleep. And if you're not well rested, forget about the vim and vigour you need to go to the gym or play a good game of tennis.

There's also a funny relationship between exercise and sleep when it comes to stress, be it financial, emotional or work-related. When you're stressed your body releases cortisol. This hormone is what's behind the 'fight-or-flight' response to danger; without it, you'd just sit there as the lion approached you. But cortisol also affects your ability to sleep. If your body is in fight-or-flight mode, it's not going to settle down for a nap, and if you are suffering from chronic stress, raised cortisol levels can interfere with sleep. On the other hand, regular exercise decreases the cortisol levels in the body, another reason why exercise helps with sleep (and why, when you are stressed, it is doubly important to get your exercise).

Clearly, the two bookends of action and inaction, though on the surface very different, are actually tethered together. And both are needed to maintain good health, with no exceptions granted.

Having said that, let's take a look at each of these bookends individually.

Keep moving

By now you know that when it comes to figuring out the best things we need to sustain good nutrition and good health, I always like to look at our evolutionary past. So the same goes for exercise.

Humans have lived in the natural world for hundreds of thousands, if not millions, of years. Our bodies evolved in lockstep with that natural world, and back then we didn't die from lifestyle-induced illnesses such as cancer or coronary disease or diabetes. We died from things like starvation, freezing, being eaten by larger animals, and, strangely enough, from infections caused by tooth decay, one of the top killers of pre-civilized man. (Hurray for modern dentists. Without them I'd be long toothless from all the sugar I consumed as a kid!)

The point is that we adapted to our world by eating in a certain way, by sleeping a certain number of hours during the night, and by walking a certain number of miles during the day. Today we are free from the constraints imposed by night and day, and from the perpetual slog of acquiring enough food. But we are not free from the patterns of behaviour imprinted in our DNA over those aeons of time.

Think about exercise this way. Our patterns of physical movement come from the fact that we are all descended from hunter-gatherers. Hunting meant that we had to do a lot of running, and use our upper-body strength for actions such as spearing, stabbing and hacking. Gathering, on the other hand, involved a lot of walking and stretching.

But the need for exercise is more than just having the equipment to walk, run and throw things. It's that, having adapted ourselves to the need for almost perpetual motion, we can't do without it. We're like cars that need to be driven, or else their engines seize up. And this is not too far off the mark. We need to exercise in order to sweat toxins from our bodies, like exhaust from an engine. We need to move in order to have healthy backbones, since nutrition and lubrication reach inside our discs only when we move our spines, in a piston-like action. We need exercise or our blood vessels don't get to dilate and then contract, instead becoming as stiff and brittle as unused rubber hoses.

There may be even more profound reasons why we need to move, having to do with the overall signals our muscles send to our brain. In our evolutionary past, we lived according to seasons. We hunted and gathered more in spring and summer than autumn and winter. Some doctors believe that when we don't exercise much, we're telling our brains that it's winter in the cave, so we should hunker down, scale back on muscle and hang on to our fat. The opposite – to build muscle and burn fat – is the message that movement sends.

The evidence that movement is good for us is incontrovertible. Study after study shows that regular exercise reduces the risk of heart disease and stroke, reduces blood pressure, helps keep body fat under control, reduces back pain and promotes bone formation. It also keeps our brains functioning at their best. One recent study by the Cleveland Clinic showed that older people who exercise moderately a few times a week have significantly less brain shrinkage than their sedentary companions, even if they are genetically predisposed to Alzheimer's.[1] This follows a Cleveland Clinic study from a few years back that showed significantly more brain activity for older folks who exercise regularly.[2]

There are literally legions of studies like these, going back to when this was big news in the 1980s and 1990s, when a lot of the groundbreaking research was done.[3] And it's not just about staying healthy as we get older. There are plenty of studies that show the benefits of regular exercise for the young. Recent research at McMaster University in Ontario showed that people of any age who exercised moderately for three hours a week had much younger and healthier skin than those who were sedentary.[4] Another study of 40,000 runners showed a much lower incidence of eye disease compared to non-runners;[5] there is also research on how exercise improves our self-esteem, reduces depression, alleviates anxiety and helps us manage stress.[6]

Overall, according to the Mayo Clinic, exercise has seven big benefits: it helps control weight, it helps fight disease, it improves our mood, it give us energy, it promotes sleep, it puts the spark back into our sex lives and it improves our happiness by getting us outdoors and helping us to connect socially.[7]

So how much?

With all these benefits stacking up – including the big benefit of improving our baseline metabolism so that we're burning more calories all day long – the big question is: how much exercise do we really need? Before answering this I must tell you my secret: I have a problem with exercise – I'm just not a big fan of it. Don't get me wrong: I love it when I'm in a routine, but as soon as I fall off the wagon and have three or four days of downtime, I really hate the start-back-up phase. I know I need to do it. When I get stressed or busy, or I'm travelling, exercise is the easiest thing for me to let go. Which makes it really hard to get started again, and doesn't help with managing my stress or getting sleep. So I need to know, how much do I really need?

To answer that, I consulted the experts, namely the folks at the US Department of Health & Human Services. They put out something called the PAG, or Physical Activity Guidelines for Americans.[8]

Here's a happy fact for me. It turns out that in terms of being healthy, what you eat is more important than exercise. You can exercise all you want, but if your fuel is wrong, you will have a hard time keeping the weight off and staying healthy. The other happy fact is that you don't have to exercise for more than half an hour a day. According to the PAG, the average adult should do at least two and a half hours of moderate intensity aerobic exercise a week, along with some muscle-strengthening activities twice a week. That's about half an hour, five days a week, or 24 minutes every day. They also point out that 10-minute blocks are good. So we're talking about two brisk 10-minute walks a day at a minimum. Not too tough.

Just for the record, aerobic activity is defined as one where people move their large muscles 'in a rhythmic manner for a sustained period'. This means that weight lifting (jerky and not sustained) doesn't count, but dancing does. Singles tennis, where you are moving pretty much continuously, is considered aerobic, whereas doubles – or golf, for that matter – is not considered aerobic because there are too many breaks where you're just standing there.

Other examples of aerobic activity include walking briskly, bicycling, swimming, rowing – you get the idea. All you have to do is keep moving.

If you want to spend even less time exercising, you just

go at it harder. The experts say you can get the same benefit in half the time from 'vigorous-intensity' aerobic activity – about 75 minutes each week if you pick up the pace. That's less than 11 minutes a day. And making it vigorous is just what it sounds like: running or jogging instead of walking; doing hard laps in the pool instead of that gentle breaststroke; playing basketball instead of badminton. Researchers found that even a few minutes of intense exercise a day – exercise that approaches your maximum capacity – produces molecular changes in your muscles that are similar to those created by several hours of light running or biking.[9]

Of course, we don't usually exercise that way, doing wind sprints for 12 minutes a day. It's more likely we'll go for a 30–40 minute run two or three times a week. The same goes for muscle strengthening. Twice a week should do it, with sessions that don't need to be more than 20 minutes or so each – stuff like weight lifting, or push-ups, or rowing, or Pilates. Remember, though, when you factor in travel time to a gym, wardrobe changes and everything else, a formal exercise regime is more like an hour a day than 20 or 30 minutes.

That's where it breaks down for me. How to handle this time commitment is one of my toughest challenges, especially since it's making time for something that I don't really want to do. Still, if I don't find a way to incorporate exercise into my life on a regular basis, I'm really going to struggle to maintain the level of happiness that I want.

This situation is kind of funny because when I was young I was very active. Australians love the beach and their sports. I played rugby in my teens and twenties, which is such a vigorous, rough exercise that the authorities are always talking about banning it. But I loved the rough-housing and didn't think of it as a sport. It was just fun, and it was social. If you ask me the best way to get exercise, I'll tell you to make it fun and social. And look for opportunities to move.

So those are really the two kinds of exercise you can get – short and vigorous (which includes weight training), or longer and easier paced. I always used to think that exercise was about taking your body to the limits of its capability. But it's also about just staying active. As usual, it goes back to our caveman days. We were either hunting, where we pushed ourselves to the limit, or gathering, where we simply moved along gradually, picking at roots, seeds, fruits and leaves.

The good thing about walking as exercise is that you can do it anywhere, and with a friend it's even better. And it's probably easier to make that part of a routine, which is what you need to do. I find that keeping up a regular practice of exercise is essential because it's so tough to get it all going again when I've been away from it. Your muscles get sore, so you don't want to do it the next day. Or worse, you overdo it (beware the Weekend Warrior!) and get hurt. Before you know it, you're calling yourself stupid, or lazy, or better off without it. So the idea is to find an exercise routine that you can maintain, not let come and go.

For me, getting back into exercise is a prime time for making excuses, something I'm really good at. My excuse is that I do a lot of travelling, which makes it hard to maintain a routine; you're tired, in different time zones, away from your regular gym. Heck, these are good excuses! On my recent book tour I probably went to 20 cities in 20 days. I had the best intentions of keeping up my exercise regime, but there were early morning calls to TV and radio stations, then press interviews, then trying to answer emails and catch up with the team in the office, then the author appearances – which always energize me – followed by a late-night meal, crashing and then getting up early. True, I could have gone for a walk after the TV interview, and I do like walking around foreign cities, but I always found something more urgent, or I was on the phone, or I was hungry. My internal dialogue and justifications for not exercising are so convincing that, if I could put that voice into the body of a lawyer, I'd win every case.

I travelled so much that I eventually asked a personal trainer friend of mine, Radan Strum, to design a series of exercises I could do in a hotel room. You can see these on the www.rebootwithjoe.com site, under the Fitness tab. We call it the Reboot Movement Method, and if you watch the videos, you can see that these are pretty straightforward exercises, both low- and high-intensity, that just about anyone can practise. Put a little music on and you're all set.

The important thing is to keep it regular, not to stop and start. The way I see it, your body has a memory. If you go a couple of years without touching your toes, it can get pretty hard. But if you've gone for two years touching your toes daily, touching them on day 731 is vastly easier than if you hadn't bothered on those previous 730 days. There is a memory to exercise, to the way your body performs and what the muscles are supposed to do.

I like to think of exercise memory as a return to youth – you bring the past into the present with you every day. At 48 years of age, I reckon I've lost a bit of memory about how I was in my twenties due to a lack of exercise over the last two decades. I don't think I can get it back to where I was then, but I'm hopeful I can get it back to where I was a decade ago. It's a lot harder to start up again, but after you've done the hard work, it's then a maintenance thing, all about holding the memory.

The big problem with holding that memory – i.e. exercising regularly – is that once you get past your excuses, you've got to find the time, and keep that time slot open. That's why some people like to exercise first thing in the morning. You wake up, get out of bed, go and do your 15 or 20 or 30 minutes. The time can't be taken away from you later by interruptions or a busy schedule, and it sets a nice tone for the whole day as well. Regardless of your best time, stick to it, because routine is really important.

A less formal approach to exercise is just to be conscious of movement, and of any opportunity for more. When you think about it, exercise as a special 'activity' is kind of a strange concept. As humans, we've been moving forever. We were always in motion, we picked up stuff, we walked somewhere, we ran somewhere else, we were always chasing this or gathering that. But because today's lifestyle is so sedentary, we need to make sure we incorporate movement whenever and wherever.

I've been in office buildings where people take the elevator to the first floor. Why not use the stairs? And what about drivers who circle parking lots in search of the closest space to the store? Better by far to park farther away and get in a few extra steps. Or what about that dinner engagement across town? I might take a cab there to be on time and not all sweaty, but afterwards I'll walk the few miles home. You'd be surprised at how these movements add up by the end of the day.

Our need for movement is so critical that OSHA, the US government agency that oversees worker safety, is now establishing guidelines for desk workers, recommending that they stand up from their chairs to stretch and walk once an hour.[10] The TV personality Dr Oz has already labelled sitting as the new smoking, and the evidence suggests that sitting for long, unbroken hours can cause havoc with our health; sit enough on the job and not even exercise after work can undo the damage. Some doctors even recommend a stretch every 20 minutes, though that seems like way too much work to me. Doing a little dance or a walkabout once an hour seems to do the trick. In fact, right now, as I finish writing this paragraph, I am going to step away from the desk and go for a 15-minute walk around the block . . .

. . . I'm back now, and it was good. It was such a beautiful day out that I actually walked for 30 minutes. So in the end, we all need to get off the couch and move around, but we also have to put things in perspective. Is your aim to get onto the set of *Baywatch*? Do you want to go ballistic and get your body fat down to 7 per cent? What I'm talking about is getting enough movement so that you'll be able to do all the things you want to do in your daily life and not be hamstrung by immobility. The degree to which you remain mobile – and flexible – is critical when it comes to feeling young. It's pretty hard to feel like a 28-year-old if you can't bend over to tie your shoelaces.

Just don't think of exercise as a dieting tool. For dieting, what you put into your body is much, much more important. If you think you're exercising as a way to lose weight, don't. It helps a lot with being healthier, but not with weight loss. In fact, strenuous exercise can increase the body's production of appetite hormones, leading people who exercise to eat even more.

And don't make exercise a chore. The only way you can sustain exercise is if it's fun, and then it's actually better for you. Earlier this year the Grenoble School of Management in France published the results of a series of social psychology experiments about exercise. Researchers asked volunteers to walk a one-mile course, after which food was served as a reward. Regardless of gender or type of snack, those volunteers who were told they would be doing 'exercise' always grumbled more and ate more. Those who were told that they were supposed to have fun and enjoy a lovely walk found the experience to be a better one, and ate less at the end.[11] Sound familiar? Guess that might be why I never thought of rugby as exercise.

And here's another good bit of information: when you start eating the right kind of food, guess what? You start to find that you want to exercise more.

And now for some sleep

Now that you've had plenty of exercise, you're ready for a good night's sleep, one of the pillars of a healthy lifestyle. Unfortunately, some of us don't find it all that easy.

One of the biggest challenges in our modern lifestyle is getting enough sleep. We try to squeeze more out of a given day by sleeping less, but even when we do finally put our head down, the quality of that rest is typically compromised by everything from the technology of our modern world to our eating and drinking habits.

Like healthy eating, everyone knows you need enough sleep. We all know how sluggish our day can be when we don't get enough. But it goes beyond that. There is a large amount of research indicating that the amount of time you sleep can affect your weight. Simply put, if you don't get enough sleep – the recommended amount is now 7–8 hours a night – you'll find it harder to lose weight and harder to keep it off.[12]

There are a number reasons why this is so. First and foremost is that people who don't get enough sleep feel tired, and they tend to fight their feelings of tiredness and fatigue by eating more. And it's not just the quantity of extra food consumed, but the quality. If you are exhausted, you're more likely to crave a sugary food for the quick burst of energy it provides.[13] This leads in short order to a sugar crash, and the need for more cheap fuel to keep the cycle going.

Beyond the sugar fix that you need to stay awake, there are deeper, more complex reasons why inadequate sleep makes it harder to lose weight or to maintain weight loss. Researchers say the length and quality of your sleep affects your hormonal activity, which is directly tied to your appetite.[14]

The two hormones that affect appetite are leptin and ghrelin. Leptin, made by your fat cells, is designed to regulate the amount of fat your body stores. When the amount reaches an adequate level, leptin is secreted and goes to your brain to inhibit the sensation of hunger. For this reason, leptin is called the 'satiety hormone' because it makes you feel satiated or full.

Ghrelin, on the other hand, is produced in the gastro-intestinal tract. When your stomach is empty, ghrelin is secreted and it tells your brain that you're hungry. Not surprisingly, it's called 'the hunger hormone'.

The classic study about how less-than-adequate sleep affects these hormones was conducted by the University of Chicago about a decade ago. Subjects who had their sleep cut to four hours a night for two nights saw an 18 per cent drop in leptin, and a whopping 28 per cent gain in ghrelin. This is why sleepless nights are normally followed by a day when, no matter what a person eats, they may not feel satisfied.[15]

The study also noted that besides an increase in appetite, the subjects craved calorie-dense, high-carbohydrate foods. The researchers were not entirely clear why sleep-deprived subjects found foods such as chocolate, cookies and cake more appealing, besides the obvious wallop of cheap energy. They postulated that the sleepy subjects were less able to think clearly and make good decisions, 'making it harder to push away the doughnuts'.

It's not just the amount of sleep that counts either. Just as important is the quality of sleep. Deep, restful, high-quality sleep plays an important role in maintaining health. Just look at people with sleep apnoea, a disorder in which the breathing stops during sleep for up to a minute at a time. This can happen scores of times during the night, so even if these individuals have put in the time, they might not be getting the benefits. And guess what? People with sleep apnoea also tend to be overweight.[16]

By the way, don't think you're alone in suffering the effects of sleep loss. In the USA at least, it's now an epidemic, and it's been building for years. Back in 1960, American adults slept an average of eight and a half hours a night. Now, over 50 years later, the average nightly sleep has fallen to less than seven hours. And the loss is most pronounced in young adults, those who are most tied to a high-tech way of life, in which the natural rhythms of sleep are wrecked by a world that is lit up and inter-connected 24 hours a day. The result is that more than three-quarters of young adults today sleep less than eight hours a night, and more than a third average less than seven.[17]

This drop in average sleep time has paralleled the explosion of American obesity. In 1960, when they were still getting enough sleep, only one in four US adults was overweight, and only about one in nine was considered obese. Today, according to the Centers for Disease Control and Prevention, more than two-thirds of US adults are overweight, and more than one in three is considered to be obese.[18] And while lack of sleep is certainly not the only cause, it's clearly one of the culprits. One study showed that people who sleep less than four hours a night are 73 per cent more likely to be obese.[19] Insufficient sleep can also cause the release of additional cortisol – the stress hormone – which can stimulate hunger.[20]

Want more research? There's plenty, but I'll give you just one additional study. This one was done at Case Western University, a study of nearly 70,000 middle-aged women over a 16-year period. What they found was that women who slept six hours a night were more likely to experience weight gain than those who slept seven hours a night. Just a one-hour difference was all it took. Granted, the difference in weight was an average of just 1.6 pounds a year, but that can add up – 16 pounds over a decade – and does make a difference.[21]

So, besides eating more to overcome sleepiness, and besides our hormones going off kilter, what else is going on with sleep loss in terms of how it affects our ability to lose weight and keep it off? If you look across the whole spectrum of studies, there are other possible factors at play:

Sleeping less . . .

. . . may cause changes in, and reduce, a person's basal metabolic rate (the number of calories you burn while at rest).

. . . interferes with the body's ability to metabolize carbohydrates and can cause high blood glucose, leading to higher insulin levels and greater body-fat storage.

. . . affects non-exercise-associated thermogenesis (involuntary activity, such as fidgeting, which generates body heat). It may be that if you sleep less, you move around less too, and therefore burn up fewer calories.

. . . means you're simply likely to have less energy during the day. Sleep more and you have more energy, are more active and eat less.

. . . impairs your judgement and adversely affects your basic discipline. You just won't care as much.

The moral, therefore, is *sleep more* if you need to, and *sleep better*. It's not just your weight that's at stake, but a whole army of health and behavioural problems.

What you can do

In the short term, sleep loss causes fatigue, lethargy, irritability, moodiness, poor cognitive function, memory impairment, increased appetite and many other symptoms that can make the simplest task feel overwhelming.

Over the longer term, poor sleep may cause significant health problems – certainly all of those associated with excess weight, such as an increased risk of diabetes, heart disease, stroke and hypertension. One study found that getting less than six hours of sleep a night was linked to a dramatically increased risk of death, especially from coronary disease.[22] Sleep deprivation has also been found to increase the risk of depression and anxiety.[23]

Getting a good night's sleep is, in fact, one of the most important things you can do for your overall health and well-being. Adequate sleep allows the body cells and tissues to repair and recover from the day. Sleep is important for the growth and rejuvenation of all the body systems – immune, nervous, skeletal, muscular . . . everything.

Remember, quality sleep is very important for weight control. People who sleep less than seven hours per night have been shown to consume an extra 500 calories per day compared to people who sleep for seven to nine hours. So rest up.[24]

TIPS FOR IMPROVING SLEEP

Ready to get a good night's sleep? Try the following:

1 **Eat right.** Eating a diet high in nutrients and minerals, particularly magnesium and calcium, will help your energy levels and encourage a better night's sleep. Dark green leafy vegetables such as kale, spinach, chard (silverbeet), Brussels sprouts, broccoli, parsley and watercress, as well as other vegetables such as celery, sweet potato and onion, are all high in calcium and magnesium. Fruit containing high amounts of these minerals are oranges, dates, figs, dried apricots, avocados and bananas.[24] This may be why most poor sleepers report drastic improvements while Rebooting.

2 **Turn off the tech.** Avoid exposure in the evenings where possible to artificial light from electronic devices, such as smartphones, iPads, computers and televisions. These will inhibit your melatonin production, which is your hormone of rest. If you use your phone as an alarm, I suggest putting it on flight mode and facing it down to avoid disturbances and radiation exposure while sleeping. If you sleep near a digital alarm clock, make sure the LED lights are red, not blue or green, as we tend to sleep better with red light.

3 **Dim the lights.** Melatonin is the natural 'sleep' hormone produced by the pineal gland each night. Not only does it help maintain our circadian rhythms – our 24-hour clock – it's also a powerful antioxidant that helps protect the nuclei and mitochondria in our DNA. In order to take advantage of this natural mechanism, avoid having too many lights on in the house in the evenings, as this will reduce your melatonin production. Lighting just a few lamps that offer a low light will help. And try never to sleep in a room where the lights are actually on!

4   Rise and shine, literally. Your natural circadian biological clock is run not only by the night's dark, which leads to the production of melatonin; exposure to natural light in the morning also supports a healthy circadian rhythm, as it signals to the hypothalamus, which controls a cascade of hormonal changes in the pituitary, pineal, adrenal and thyroid glands. It also affects the immune system. So keep your days bright and your nights dark.

5   Set the mood. Your sleep area should be dark with plenty of ventilation. It should be an oasis of rest. Don't associate it with other activities, such as playing video games. Pavlov knew what he was doing with his dogs. Make your bed the bell that says it's time to sleep, not play.

6   Stay on schedule. Trying to go to bed at the same time every night will promote a regular sleep time. This goes back to the circadian rhythms. We are creatures of daily routine, so if you go to bed at a certain hour each night, and wake at a certain hour each day, these habits tend to form neural patterns that are easier to maintain than random times for sleeping and rising.

7   Know the golden hours. The optimum hours for true regenerative sleep are between 10pm and 3am. Remember the expression 'every hour before midnight is worth two after midnight'. Yes, this seems a little early, especially if you are young and want to catch a gig that starts at 10.30pm. Make these excursions the exception, not the rule, and you'll get better, deeper sleep.

8   No booze, more snooze. Alcohol is a common 'cure' for insomnia – in fact, doctors once recommended 'nightcaps' to help with sleep – but drinking before bedtime, while it may induce drowsiness, leads to poor-quality sleep by disrupting sleep stages and causing abrupt awakenings during the night. Most people don't realize this, but they have tossed and turned all night. So avoid alcohol several hours before going to bed.

9 **Keep your plate light at night.** Avoid eating heavy evening meals. Your digestive system slows down when you sleep, and a full stomach will result in a restless night. This is especially true if it's a spicy meal, which can lead to heartburn. Try to eat about three or four hours before bed, and make your evening meal a light to moderate meal. Foods that contribute to a good night's sleep are rich in tryptophan, a sleep-promoting substance found in nuts, seeds, bananas, honey, eggs and, most famously, in turkey and warm milk.

10 **Cut the caffeine.** Everyone metabolizes caffeine differently, and some people are more tolerant of its effects than others. But caffeine is a stimulant that people drink to wake up. Therefore, caffeinated beverages should be avoided in the evening if you want good sleep. The obvious culprits are coffee, tea and cola, but caffeine is also found in drinks and desserts containing cocoa, as well as the ultimate expression of cocoa, chocolate. Preferably avoid all these things after 2pm.

11 **Inhale, exhale.** Use essential oils such as lavender, geranium, chamomile, rose and others in oil burners, in baths, or in a spritzer mixed with water around your sleep area. Or you can add a few drops to your shower floor as you're having a hot shower. According to research at Ruhr University in Germany, jasmine is as potent as the drug Valium when it comes to its soothing effect, which acts on the receptors for GABA in nerve and organ cells. (GABA is a neurotransmitter that has a calming effect on the brain.)

12 **Exercise, but not too late.** Daily exercise is one of the traditional solutions for deep, restful sleep, especially if you have a sedentary job or lifestyle. According to a study by the National Sleep Foundation, 150 minutes of moderate to vigorous exercise a week (about 20 minutes a day) delivers a 65 per cent improvement in sleep quality.[25] Just try not to exercise within two hours of your bedtime as this will stimulate your heart rate and metabolism and disrupt restful sleep.

13 **Rest, relax and wind down.** Many sleep specialists will tell you that anxiety is the number one cause of insomnia, so practise calm activities for at least an hour before bed, such as reading a book, taking a bath, writing, knitting, drawing or meditating. News reports, stimulating television programmes or suspenseful movies can interfere with a restful night. Another trick is to keep a 'worry journal', where you record your biggest concerns for the next day and how you're going to deal with them, even if it's just a note to think about it more tomorrow. Gets them off your chest.

14 **Drink less liquid.** If you have a tendency to need the toilet during the night, avoid drinking one or two hours before bed. While it's very important to stay well hydrated during the day and early evening, after about 8pm you should be tapering off. Good, uninterrupted sleep will elude you if you have to get up to go to the bathroom in the middle of the night.

15 **Sip to soothe.** If you're going to drink before bed, consume herbal teas, such as chamomile, lemon balm, passionflower, limeflower, valerian and other restful blends. A chamomile-lavender mixture is good, for the reasons mentioned earlier about lavender's properties as a scent. And then there's always warm milk, which can be enhanced with some honey (tryptophan) and a dash of nutmeg (tranquillizing chemical compounds).

16 **Don't worry about the sleep itself.** An interesting bind that people get into is not being able to sleep because they are worrying about their inability to sleep. There is a certain, perverse wish-fulfilment going on here. Instead of thinking about something else, or even about the joy of a good night's sleep, you think about the horrors of continued insomnia. You can overcome this with positive thinking, deep breathing and letting go. Or you can read a book for a while to take your mind off things. (You'll feel better anyway that you're learning something instead of stewing in the dark.)

17 **If you can't get enough, take a nap.** According to one study, a group of pilots who slept for six hours or less for seven nights while on duty found that their cortisol (stress hormone) levels increased significantly and stayed elevated for two days. The recommended seven hours of nightly shut-eye allows your body enough time to recover from the day's stress. When you fall short of the mark, take a nap the next day – Pennsylvania State University researchers found that a midday snooze cut cortisol levels by 50 per cent in subjects who'd lost sleep the previous night.

18 **Blow the long horn.** OK, this is not entirely serious, but being from Australia, I just had to mention it. You know that long horn the Aborigines blow? It's called the didgeridoo. One Australian study showed that if you blew it for 25 minutes a day, six days a week, it would improve sleep apnoea symptoms. It has something to do with strengthening the muscles around the airways.

Now, go and get a good night's sleep. Sweet dreams (pun intended)!

Sustaining a healthy lifestyle for Barry Jacinto means keeping busy – with the food and exercise log he keeps every day, with the gym he goes to four or five times a week, and with the time he spends carefully preparing each meal.

'I just make myself busy, to get into it every day,' says Barry, who weighed 23½ stone (330 pounds) when he did his first Reboot, and now weighs 13 stone (180 pounds). 'Rain or shine, I go to the gym, even if there's a snowstorm.'

He also keeps a meticulous paper log of everything he eats, and the estimated calories. As for his food, it's a plant-based diet that includes fish for protein: 'I actually love to make my own food. I love to cook and make it look beautiful.'

Mostly, however, what keeps Barry going is the satisfaction he gets from what he's accomplished for himself, and the momentum it's built for his 'journey' of personal growth and change.

'Just looking at my old picture makes me feel better for the whole day,' says the 22-year-old. 'I will watch old videos of myself and I will cry. I don't care who's in front of me, I randomly cry because I didn't know I was that big. I didn't see myself like that. I didn't know what it was to be healthy.'

He's also won kudos from the gym where he works out, which posted pictures of him and a story about his juicing. And he gets lots of feedback from his Facebook page and the online communities at www.rebootwithjoe.com.

'I get a lot of messages like,"Hey, can you help me?" I give them tips, they do it and they feel better,' says Barry. 'It's so funny how they ask me questions, because I'm not used to it. *I* used to ask people questions, now they're asking *me*. It makes me feel special.' He also shares recipes and photos of his meals. 'I post everything on Instagram and people like it, so I get a lot of messages like, "Can you cook for me?"'

When Barry started his first Reboot, he says he didn't get a lot of support from friends and relatives. 'My friends just thought I was playing around when I told them I was going to do a juicing [reboot]. They said I was crazy, you can't do that,' he says. 'So I just ignored what they said and did what was in my mind . . . As for my family, I was raised mostly by my grandma, and grandmas love food and just want you to eat.'

It wasn't until he lost 7 stone (100 pounds) that his friends came around, says Barry. 'They were surprised and now *they* want to do it.' Before then, however, he had a hard time going out with them. 'My friends would be eating chicken wings and ribs, so instead of watching them I'd walk out. I would just walk around the block, just to stay away from it.'

Today Barry takes his inspiration from friends he's made at two gyms, one where he works and another where he works out. 'They make me feel like I need to be healthy and get toned because everyone you work with in the gym is in good shape. It's not that you want to be like them, it's that you want to do better, so you can see yourself in a better way when you look in the mirror.'

As for advice to fellow travellers on the path to healthy living, Barry emphasizes the following:

First, pay attention to diet above exercise. 'It's not really about working out at the gym, it's what you eat. If you don't eat right, what's the point of going to the gym? And never go food shopping when you're hungry.'

Next, get out of your old patterns with some new activities. 'I tell people to do something new, something different. Like join some classes that you've never done before. Don't just stay on one thing. If you don't try something new, you'll never know what you might be missing.'

Most important, however, is to care about yourself. 'You've just got to love yourself, because if you don't love yourself, you can't help yourself. That's what I always say,' he says. 'My hashtag is #respectyourself.'

6
PRACTISE MINDFULNESS
(Chill Out)

We now know that a lot of eating is emotional. If you've been doing the things I've suggested, you'll have identified specifically how you are an emotional eater. What are your happy food memories? What are the foods you reach for when you're feeling the need for comfort? You've thought about what diet is good for you, how best to set yourself up with healthy habits around food, and what sort of exercise and sleep you need. You may be sailing along smoothly in your journey to health. Or maybe you're stalled and frustrated, wondering 'Why can't I do this?'

The number one reason we don't do what we know we should do – and in most cases want to do – is stress. Financial stress, emotional stress, time stress.

Let's face it – unless you live off the grid on some magical island, your life is filled with stress. It's in your job, your family and your relationships. It's the pressure to perform, to succeed, to make money, to get ahead, to win the rat race. It's in the choices you constantly have to make. It's in your responsibilities to earn money, to excel at work, to get good grades, to look attractive, or to get somewhere on time. And it's unrelenting.

We feel pressure to find the time to take care of our parents, our children, our employees, our houses, our friends. Taking care of ourselves falls way down on the list of priorities.

Stress is also everywhere. As if our own personal problems weren't enough, our modern world kicks in with a constant bombardment from phones, iPads, desktops, laptops, television, radio, billboards, texts, Twitter, Facebook, Linked In, Pinterest, streaming video – it goes on and on, with more to come, such as wristwatch computers and the iGlass. Even the cars and planes that once offered a brief oasis are now equipped with video screens, phones and wi-fi connectivity. Take a cab in New York and you're watching TV news in the back seat instead of enjoying the city views. We are now supposed to be always available, and we are always distracted. It's incredibly stressful.

In and of itself, stress is not bad. It's the mechanism behind the fight-or-flight response, the tool that helped us survive as humans. Out on the savannah, stress kept us alive by jump-starting our bodies whenever we faced a threat. Sudden danger? Our adrenal system flooded us with hormones such as cortisol, which got our hearts pumping and our energy soaring, shutting down non-essential things like digestion and ramping up things like the flow of glucose and oxygen to our muscles.

The problem is that while short-term stress is good, long-term stress is a killer. If there is one thing that virtually all doctors agree on, it's that chronic stress is harmful. It leads to all sorts of trouble, like a weakened immune system that leaves you open to colds and viruses, or circulatory overload that causes high blood pressure and strokes. The list goes on from there. Chronic stress contributes to diabetes, heart problems, cancer, arthritis, anxiety, depression, insomnia and poor sleep, headaches and poor digestion. Stress, except when you need it to fight or flee, is just not healthy for us – it's estimated that 75–90 per cent of all visits to the doctor are for stress-related complaints.[1]

Most people try to deflect stress by self-medicating with foods that are full of sugar, fat and salt, or with drugs, cigarettes and alcohol. For years I used all these things to deal with my super-high levels of stress, which I reckon I lived with for most of my adult life.

I started out on the Sydney Futures Exchange, a high-stress environment of buying and selling, where I risked making or losing tens of thousands of dollars a day. (It's no wonder that lunch for all the traders was washed down with a lot of booze.) That stress increased when I began investing in and starting companies; there was always the chance of making a ton of money – or of going bankrupt.

I think the first time in my adult life that I actually de-stressed for any length of time was when I filmed *Fat, Sick & Nearly Dead*. Drinking juice and driving across the USA, I had no worries, no other commitments, and all the time I needed. But after the Reboot, when I was back under financial stress – this time to get the movie out and pay my team – and I was under relationship stress, the cortisol was pumping overtime. This meant I wasn't sleeping well, so during the day, tired, I'd want quick energy from sugar. And because I was tired, I didn't have as much will-power to make the right choices. Instead of resisting the urge for a quick fix, I'd give in 'just this once'! (Remember Phil's 'OK tos?')

The fact is that when we're stressed we go right to emotional eating, we crave our comfort foods and we make bad choices – and that stresses us out even more. It's a vicious cycle, and it knocks us off our game. Let's face it: if you're stressed out, you're going to have a hard time following any of the advice in this book.

So how can we deal with this monster called stress? How can we avoid turning to processed foods and chemicals that deal only with the symptoms, resulting in something even worse later on? In a word: mindfulness.

Tune in, calm down

Mindfulness, and the ability to relax that mindfulness gives you, is a vital tool in sustaining a healthy life. As just noted, one of the main reasons we slide back into our old habits is stress. How much better if we were able to find the place inside that lets us take a deep breath and relax, and gain some perspective and self-control – allowing us to know *and* to do?

It's little wonder, then, that mindfulness is a growing movement in many Western nations – an antidote to the poisonous tsunami of stress and stimulus overload. People are looking for some way to unplug and decompress. And I would have to agree: mindfulness has never been more important in our human history than it is today. This is especially true when it comes to sustaining healthy habits of eating, exercise and sleep. We are hammered by our own personal stress, then bounced around like pinballs in a giant marketing maze, pushed and pulled by the seductions of bliss points and processed foods, by cues that induce over-eating and by the sheer distractions of the modern world that keep us off our game. Mindfulness is an important tool to return the power of self-control to the user, which is us.

But just what is mindfulness?

The definition I like is that mindfulness is a state of calm awareness, of paying attention to the present moment with such focus that it's impossible to worry about anything else. It's really a time-out, and therefore a chance to de-stress.

You may be familiar with meditation, which is a kind of mindfulness. I guess like 'vegan', some people like to dress up meditation as a lifestyle, with new-age, hippyish trappings about chakras, crystals and wearing purple. Now that might be ok if you're a fan of purple, but for an Australian bloke like me, mindfulness is just an easier word to swallow. I also think meditation is more formal, a programme to follow. There are many ways we can be mindful without formally sitting down to meditate. Prayer is a form of mindfulness, going for walk in a quiet place can be a form of mindfulness. Long-distance runners sometimes describe their runs as 'zen-like' – they run without headphones, a steady breathing in and out, and have no idea what they thought about for the whole time.

So you don't need to formally meditate to be mindful, not that I have any objections to meditation. I have friends who practise meditation 15–30 minutes a day – transcendental meditation, guided meditation, yogic meditation, 'tapping' – and I think it's great for them. Dozens of studies, many funded by the US National Institute of Health, have shown that meditation is an effective tool for alleviating high blood pressure, depression and anxiety.[2] Even the American Heart Association is now on board, advocating transcendental meditation for reducing atherosclerosis, constriction of blood vessels (which causes high blood pressure), and thickening of the coronary arteries.[3]

However, I am not going to presume to teach you to meditate. Why? I don't have a meditation practice. I'm trying, but I'm just not very good at it. I'm the relentless sort, an all or nothing kind of guy. When I'm stressed, my reaction is to press on the accelerator. So I've looked for other ways to be mindful.

If you are interested in meditation, there are many good sites, such as www.headspace.com and www.deepakchopra.com. One of the easiest and most effective techniques (maybe because it's easy!) is something that our friend, author and healer Abdi Assadi teaches the folks who attend our Camp Reboot. Deep breathing. You'd be surprised how shallow most of us breathe, just using the top half of our lungs.

What Abdi teaches is that you need to breathe from the abdomen, opening up the lower sections of the lungs. This is the kind of deep breathing we do when we sleep. If you pay attention to your breathing, and breathe slowly and deeply, you'll be amazed by how much you are able to relax. And it doesn't have to be a big deal. If you can set aside 10 minutes a day to sit quietly and pay attention to your breathing, you'll make some real progress (and you'll be meditating, by the way).

Abdi has a specific technique he teaches – head slightly down, tongue at the top of the teeth/bottom of the gum, index fingers pointing down, slightly up on the toes, breathing in and out through the nose 10 times. Do this when you're queueing at the bank, or waiting to board an aircraft, or being jostled in the deli. It's amazing how relaxing this exercise is. (If you want more pointers, check out the video of Abdi teaching me to meditate on www.rebootwithjoe.com/abdi.)

Again, part of the idea of paying attention to your breathing is to take your mind off your thoughts. You can't be anxious about something if you're not thinking about it. So anything you can do to stop thinking about your problems, even if just for a little while, acts like a tonic. This is one of the reasons music makes us happy. It helps us escape the gnarly bonds of thought, and all that implies – including negativity, doubt and worry.

This is not as easy as it may sound, by the way. In his book *The Power of Now*, Eckhart Tolle points out how powerful thought has become in our modern world, how it rules us and how we can't control it. Just try sitting calmly in a quiet place and letting your mind empty out. What you will find, just as I did, is that thoughts pop up from nowhere, bubble to the surface, or creep in from all sides, like snakes. It's just incredibly hard to turn that part of your brain off.

Mindfulness is indeed a powerful tool, because when you are in a state of mindfulness you can observe your thoughts and feelings from a distance, without being caught up in them and without judging them. As Abdi Assadi likes to point out, thinking and food are both things that we use to numb ourselves, and both can be as addictive as drugs.

Each person, however, has to find his or her best path to mindfulness; it's not the same for all of us. As I said, I'm still learning and finding my way with meditation. I have been practising yoga lately and I'm really enjoying that. I like having an instructor telling me what to do because I have to think even less. Besides quieting your mind, yoga is also a great way to stretch your muscles and keep yourself flexible, especially your spine.

For others, mindfulness may be as simple as taking a long walk in the woods and paying attention to nature instead of the commotion in their head. For me, having lived near the ocean most of my life, it's a walk on the beach. Nothing beats the sound of crashing waves and the smell of salty air to make me feel relaxed and refreshed. And if you can't find time during the day to carve out a window of relaxed awareness, you should consider starting and ending each day with a little session of mindfulness.

Taming the triggers

If you do practise mindfulness on a regular basis, whether through long walks in nature, deep breathing, or a daily meditation, you'll find you can relax more easily when faced with stress throughout the day. Anchoring your day with periods of mindfulness has a kind of calming effect on the rest of the time. You're just more relaxed.

Still, dealing with stress is not just a matter of reducing the overall level of anxiety that permeates our lives. It's also a matter of dealing with the sudden onset of stressful events, the triggers that set us off.

At the end of the day, what you have to ask yourself is, 'Where does all the stress come from?' I think a lot of it stems from ourselves. The trigger may come from the outside, but doesn't the stress really come from us, what we put on ourselves with our response? Sure, a lot of our troubles, such as financial concerns, come from external sources. But, as often as not, it's our reaction to things that raises the level of stress.

For sustaining a healthy lifestyle, mindfulness is a great tool for overall de-stressing. But it's also a tool to defuse the kind of behaviours that lead us back to bad habits. You know the old expression, 'Just take a deep breath' when you're faced with distressing news? That adage is basically good advice on how to avoid what is called 'reactive' behaviour.

We all have a tendency to overreact to incoming stimuli, often before we even think about them. We even have a phrase for it – a 'knee-jerk reaction' – which refers to what happens when a doctor whaps your leg right below the kneecap with a little rubber mallet. This is to test whether your nerves are in good shape and react automatically.

This kind of physical reaction is based on an immediate, closed loop that never reaches your conscious mind. It just happens, like it's out of your control. This is the kind of reactive behaviour behind a lot of violence. People react without thinking. It's the cooler heads that prevail, which means taking a step back and looking at the situation with a little more wisdom than just smacking someone in the face.

When it comes to poor eating habits, reactive behaviour plays a big part. Food vendors know and use this. I don't know about you, but when I find myself reaching for that chocolate bar at the checkout counter, it's not because I'm in a really happy mood or feeling great about myself; it's because I'm terribly frustrated. I just waited at the bank for 20 minutes because they wanted me to sign something, and I've probably waited another 10 minutes at this checkout, which means I won't have time to exercise this morning, and I keep getting emails from people at the office about things that need my attention . . . I want that chocolate! So what if I just lower my head slightly, stop looking at the brownie, breathe in and out deliberately a few times? You know what, I feel more relaxed, and suddenly that chocolate isn't quite so urgent.

Mindfulness lets you take a step back, even if just for a moment, and this helps big-time in how you react to food. And that's something that mindfulness gives you: a bit of perspective; another handle on dealing with the chain-reaction of stress.

Someone asked me recently how to resist certain temptations. As discussed earlier, the answer is complicated. It's a mix of establishing new habits, of re-educating your taste buds, and of feeling good and confident about yourself. But in the immediate moment of the stimulus, it comes down to separating yourself from the reactive moment, at least long enough for you to think about what you're doing. Mindfulness can give you that distance.

Even if you decide to indulge yourself once in a while, and have that special food that makes you happy, let it be your decision, made in a calm, mindful way rather than in a reckless reaction to stress. This is something we'll talk about in the final chapter. But for now, think of it this way: make it a knowing decision, so that 'knowing and doing' are one.

Simplify, simplify

Beyond the overall de-stressing it provides, and the space you need to avoid brainless reactions to food and to emotional eating, mindfulness is also a way to deal with a world full of noise. As we all know, technology is just going to become more and more invasive. It used to be lots easier to get away from it all. Now mobile devices stick to us like bloodhounds, and it's considered almost rude not to be available via text and voice all the time.

The result of being so connected is that we are slaves to an incoming barrage of phone calls, emails, texts, tweets, instant messages, entertainment options, and so forth. This is yet another source of stress in our lives.

A lot of airtime has been given to the concept of multitasking, which for years was all the rage. The idea was that you could get several things done at the same time. It was considered the hallmark of the modern worker, though the quintessential image remains that of the mother holding her infant in one hand and a phone in the other, while simultaneously cooking dinner. We admire that sort of ability to cope with overload.

The problem with multi-tasking is that it doesn't let you concentrate on any particular project.[4] Can you imagine how our greatest writers and artists would have fared if constantly interrupted? Even though focusing on one thing at a time is what really allows us to do something well, we want technology to help us extend our tentacles in multiple directions all at once. The result is that our time gets ever more splintered as we stay in touch with our offices while on holiday, or take business calls while at home, or deal with personal issues while at work, or, worst of all, text someone else while spending time with a friend.

The point is that, while it may be hard to simplify our complex lives, we need to take the time to truly be with others and ourselves. That means turning off the TV, the phone, the computer and being available and present in the moment. Believe me, I know how tough this is. I travel all the time. I constantly feel the need to touch base with employees who are usually in a different time zone, or keep channels open if someone is reaching out for help. If I turn off the phone, the emails, texts and voice messages pile up to a point that becomes unmanageable. I actually had to take a holiday – my first in three years – just to find the time to work on this book. I had to learn to step back and unplug.

The big picture

So far, the examples of mindfulness have related to its use as a tool in daily life, to sidestep stress by paying attention to the moment and to your actions in a given day. But there is a bigger sense of mindfulness, which is to put your whole life into perspective. The purpose of this mindfulness is to look at the big picture.

Without resorting to the idea of multi-tasking, I do think you can look at the art of living as a juggling act. We all have to juggle very different aspects of our lives, but I think they boil down to five basic things: health, self, family/friends, career and love.

I find myself juggling those five things in the same way we all do – trying to find the right balance and to do my best with each one of these categories.

If you leave any one of them unattended for too long, it can pull everything down. If you let your health go, for example, what effect will that have on your ability to love and be loved? If you let your love go, what effect will that have on your self-esteem? If you let your self-esteem go, what effect will that have on your career? If your career goes, what effect can that have on family and friends?

These important aspects of life are all interconnected, and you have to be aware of that bigger picture. It's not just about eating mostly plants, or having to go for a walk around the block every day. You're like a gardener tending to multiple needs for growth, from soil to water to sunshine, to make sure that your garden will thrive. There is a mindfulness to understanding the connections between the fundamental components of a healthy life and how one aspect can have repercussions on the others.

Being mindful of the fundamentals for a healthy life can also avoid a lot of stress. If you can attend to a major category that's been ignored, and give it the attention it needs, it's less likely to crash into another part of your life and throw you off the rails. Act badly towards family and friends, for example, and that sends you down a rabbit hole of depression, which can lead to binge-eating. This sort of ultra-mindfulness can have a real knock-on effect so that you're present and aware and not making poor life choices. As Dr Ornish points out, you can't ignore an important aspect of your life, like family and friends, and think that it won't impact your overall balance.

I think that's a big part of what mindfulness does: in addition to giving us a handle to deal with stress, it brings perspective to our lives.

TIPS FOR BECOMING MINDFUL

Here are some ideas for getting the full benefits of mindfulness:

1 **Practise.** Pick a mindful exercise – deep breathing, yoga, meditation – then spend 10 minutes a day practising it. One easy way is simply to pick a time and a quiet place, and sit on a chair (or cross-legged on a cushion) and pay attention to your breath. As thoughts enter your head, don't overreact. Just observe them, then return to your focus.

2 **Wear a wristwatch.** This allows you to check the time without consulting your phone, which may take you down another rabbit hole of distraction.

3 **Turn it off.** Pick 30 minutes a day when you will turn off your phone and computer. An easy time is while you are eating lunch or dinner, but try it during your 'busy' times too.

4 **Be early.** Try arriving 15 minutes early at all your events. This will reduce a lot of operational, last-minute stress in your life. It will also give you time to relax and be more mindful about the upcoming event.

Self-awareness is the most powerful tool you can use, says Canadian Kate Elinsky. At age 55, when she started her Reboot, she bought a loose-leaf binder with 800 pages in it. When we talked to her, she had filled in 500 pages of it, one day at a time. She had also lost 12½ stone (180 pounds) and stopped all her medications for diabetes.

'It's been 500 days of having at least two juices a day,' says Kate, who lives in a small town east of Vancouver. 'I write down everything I eat, what I drink, what I weigh, my blood sugar levels, all my exercises, and what I feel emotionally. So if I had some trouble last week – perhaps I didn't lose weight, or I wasn't feeling right – I can go back and see exactly what I did that threw me off track.'

It's a matter of being 'constantly aware' says Kate, who started to juice in April 2013, five days after she saw *Fast, Sick & Nearly Dead*. 'I find that if I don't keep track of things and just start playing it by ear, I go way off. So many people give all these excuses about why they don't want to write things down and be aware of what's going on. I think, "That's OK, but that's the reason you lost 50 pounds and then gained 65 back."'

Another part of her dedication to honest self-awareness is her 'Katie Jay' blog on www.rebootwithjoe.com, and the online groups there to which she belongs. 'For me it's a daily thing. I get up, I monitor my blood sugar, I have my juice, and then I check in online to see how everybody is doing in my groups. And then I comment on how they are doing.'

That kind of regular support, she says, is critical. 'It's massively important to keep up the contact . . . There are support groups where if a person quits, it's because they've fallen off the wagon and don't want to admit that they had a really bad experience. They just don't come back.'

What Kate likes to do is keep it real, and to share that.

'There are times I go online and say, "I'm so mad at myself because I gave in to the monster and this is what happened." I have a teenage daughter, and a husband who suffers short-term memory loss. My frustration level gets so high that sometimes I can't take it any more and I just mindlessly eat. I tell them that this is what happened, and people come on and say, "Thank you for saying that." It's not all peaches and cream, and it's not happy, happy, happy all the time.'

What Kate sees are people who join the online communities with great enthusiasm, talking about their early successes. 'A week later they've quit writing and they never come back. And I know exactly why – they don't want to say I had a really hard time. They don't ask, "What can I do to make it better?" They just give up. And it breaks my heart because they don't have to. Because the support is there. There is even a nutritionist they can talk to.'

Another big tool in Kate's arsenal is her new habit of physical activity. Her small town is situated in a valley, with all kinds of opportunities to take long nature walks.

'I used to start to go for a walk with my husband, and after the first half-block I'd be out of breath and bent over, trying to ease the pain in my lower back,' she says. 'It was really a chore to go for a short walk – and that would be on a flat, level surface.' These days she likes Nordic pole-walking, which is like cross-country skiing without the skis or the snow. And she can walk to the top of hills without getting out of breath.

'When my daughter and I went to the gym the other day, she said she saw someone out of the corner of her eye on the rowing machine, and had to take a second look, because she didn't realize it was me. I said, "Want to see what I can really do?" I went on the treadmill and started running. And she started crying. She said, "Mom, I can't believe it." Because she has grown up with a morbidly obese person.'

Today Kate keeps a photo of herself on the wall next to her fridge, from the day she began to juice at 29 stone (408 pounds). 'A lot of people talk about how they absolutely hate their before picture. I think, "How in the world can I hate that girl in the picture?" She was a lot stronger than anyone gave her credit for. She fought every day so that I could survive and become who I am today.'

7
RESPECT YOURSELF (Stop Beating Yourself Up)

I've waited until this final chapter to talk about your relationship with yourself for the simple reason that it's the most important thing of all, the foundation for everything else.

Unil now, all the advice in this book has been about the tools you can use to sustain a healthy life. You need to employ these tools: knowing what a good diet is; how to have a healthy relationship with food and maintain good food habits; understanding your need for community, exercise and sleep; and learning how to be mindful and avoid stress. All are useful for building a healthier you.

In the end, however – in the all-important long run – none of these will work if you don't have a good relationship with yourself. It's that simple.

I often think to myself that I have all the knowledge I need to be supremely successful in life. I know about everything I should be doing – all the ways I should take care of my health, all the ways I should act in relationships, all the ways I should be managing my money, all the ways I should act towards my family, all the ways I should act towards myself, and so on. I know everything I need to do. So what's the problem? Me. I am the problem and the problem is me. If I could just get myself out of the way, life could be nearly perfect. I'm what's slowing down the Joe Cross Express, and I know it.

I think most people also know this – that we are our biggest hurdles. If we could just get ourselves out of the way, we could leap tall buildings in a single bound. But we don't. Whether it starts from that morning conversation of putting ourselves down, or from making promises to ourselves and then breaking them, or from setting goals that are too hard to achieve and then punishing ourselves for failing to reach them, or from being too critical about the size of our bellies or hips, of from looking at the lines in our face and not understanding that ageing is a natural part of life – we are our own worst cheerleaders. We are amazingly pessimistic about ourselves, and a lot of the negative things we experience we bring upon ourselves.

So why aren't we kinder to ourselves? Well, maybe we don't respect ourselves enough.

This thing called love

The most overused word in the English language is 'love', and it's a word that can mean a lot of different things. I can't possibly decipher all those meanings here, but when I talk about the need to respect ourselves, I think most people would call that self-love.

I reckon if you ask people whether they love themselves, and they have enough time to contemplate the question, most would answer that they do. But when you look at their actions and subconscious thought patterns, I think you could build a strong case to show that they don't. At the very least, people don't act that way. Most of us behave in ways that are negative and self-sabotaging, pulling the wings off the 'higher angels of our nature'.

The truth is that the relationship is far from black or white. We don't either hate or love ourselves all the time. I don't think anyone walks around 24/7 despising themselves. They wouldn't last too long if they did. And when it comes to loving ourselves, I think there are times when we do and times when we don't. I know there are times I certainly don't love myself (I'm not that good yet, though I'm trying to be). The important thing is to recognize the times when you don't, and then to pull out some of the tricks for loving yourself again.

Oddly enough, how we go about loving ourselves more – even just the idea of loving yourself – is not talked about a whole lot. It's certainly something we're not taught in school or college, and it's not the focus of most religions.

Yet, as discussed at the beginning of this book, the relationship we have with ourselves is the most important relationship we have. It's who we speak to the most, it's who we hang out with the most. It's there from the very beginning and to the very end. And if you don't have a good relationship with yourself – if you don't love or respect yourself – it's not going to be a fun ride.

So what does loving yourself come down to? What does the word 'love' mean, anyway? Hordes of poets and songwriters have had a stab at that for centuries. For me, it's a combination of respect, honour and care, all applied honestly. I say 'honestly' because you've got to love yourself for the right reasons – not because of the size of your bank account or the genetic blessing of good cheekbones, but for the unique spirit that makes you who you really are, underneath all the trappings of possessions and appearance.

The easier path, the mystery voice

Now, it's not always easy to respect, honour and care for yourself because you see yourself with all your faults. And when you start getting really honest with yourself, it's pretty easy to go down a black hole. It would take me a mere 10 minutes to think up enough negatives to send me into free-fall.

Having said that, I don't believe that hating ourselves is the natural state. I think if you grew up in a jungle and were really on your own Robinson Crusoe-style, you would have very few negative thoughts. If that's the case (though it's a little hard to test this one), negative thoughts must come from outside ourselves.

Once again, I'm baffled by the fact that the importance of loving and respecting ourselves is absent from our lessons at school, and even at church. But it goes farther than that. I think we are taught literally not to love ourselves, with a serving of negativity on the side.

Lots of us were raised by parents who taught us the lessons of life in a negative voice – the 'do this or else' approach. In school we are ranked and taught that someone did better or that we did worse. Christianity is all about receiving the grace of God's love when we are not worthy. In the Catholic tradition, which is how I was raised, you confess your sins and imperfections; you don't tell the priest about all the good things you've done. And the schoolyard is a training ground for negativity, where children pick on each other for any little difference, whether it's because you talk funny, have crooked teeth, big ears or a large behind.

I think this helps explain one of the great mysteries about self-hate versus self-love: where does that negative voice inside our head come from? You know the one I mean. The one that says you're not good enough, that you don't deserve success, that you're a failure and a loser. Is it the voice of your father telling you that you'll never amount to anything? Is it the voice of a world that's said 'no' so often you've absorbed it into yourself? Is it a reprimand because you're not as successful as someone else?

If you ask me, I think a big reason we're so awash in negativity is that we're brought up that way, and that we end up internalizing these voices. Plus, it's simply a lot easier to be negative than positive. It's easier to knock something down than to build it up, or to do nothing than to do something, even in the face of danger or evil.

Consequently, the journey to self-respect and self-love can be tough. It takes courage. You have to get into the house of mirrors, to look at who you really are, and to respect what you find there. It also takes work because you've got to watch yourself, catch yourself, and be conscious of what you do and say.

Be kind to others

Schoolkids can be the worst tormentors, but often adults aren't much better when it comes to tearing other people down. When I was at the height of my post-Reboot weight gain – stressed by the prospect of laying off my new team, who had all quit well-paid jobs to join me because they believed in Reboot – I was really stung by Facebook comments like, 'Hey, Joe! You're looking fat!' It made me think of how a heavier woman must feel when she hears comments like, 'You'd be so pretty if you just lost some weight!'

Why do people feel the need to make these comments? Maybe they're trying to be helpful. But guess what? Telling an overweight person they are overweight doesn't help them. It just reinforces the negative voice.

More often than not, I don't think these comments are meant to be helpful. I reckon the commenters have a strong, negative internal voice, and being negative towards someone else makes them feel better; pointing out someone else's imperfections makes *them* a little less imperfect.

Realize that everybody is struggling. Everyone on the planet has good days and bad days; everyone has problems and no one is immune. All marriages and businesses and friendships go through ups and downs. Everyone has a negative internal voice, some stronger than others.

So here's my first rule. Be kind to others. Guess what? When you start being kind to others, they are usually kind back, and that kindness helps boost your self-esteem. And a funny thing happens when you stop your negative external voice: it dampens that negative internal voice.

There is also a nice symmetry to this first step. Since a lot of negativity comes from the outside, you can start to reverse it on the outside as well.

Self-respect means self-nourishment

Being kind to others is a good start, and a good way to start changing the energy around you. What's next is even more important. If you ask me what's the crucial action you need for self-respect and self-love, I'd have to say it is to nurture yourself.

Acts of nurturing mean taking time for yourself. Granted, this is hard to do in a time-stressed world. But it can be as simple as giving yourself 15 minutes of rest and deep breathing, or going for a walk in a beautiful place, or letting yourself get a good night's sleep. I think that nourishment is very close to nurturing, so look after yourself by putting lots of fresh water into your system, and lots of fresh fruits and veggies of course.

These are things your body is craving, and if you give them to your body, the karma is immediate; your body will thank you by performing better. There is also a 'dance' here between the physical self and the spiritual or emotional self.

Another part of nurturing is how you talk to yourself. Think about how you would treat somebody you love and respect. I believe that telling them how wonderful they are would be among the first things you'd do.

Respecting yourself means positive thinking

When you beat yourself up, take a dim view of yourself and put yourself down, it's a private tirade that no one else hears but you. And like anything else in life, if you hear it enough, you start to believe it. And once you believe in it, bang! You're a goner. If you believe you're a failure, you become one.

The good news is that the opposite is equally true. As soon as you start to tell yourself you're not a failure, that you're going to do your best, and that tomorrow will be better than today, then boom! It will start to happen. This is the wonder of optimism: that if we tell ourselves good things will come our way, and we believe it, this actually helps them to take place.

One of the best-selling books of all time is *The Power of Positive Thinking* by Norman Vincent Peale. Written 75 years ago, it was among the first true self-help books. The message was that thought becomes reality, and that if you tell yourself you are a terrific and deserving person every day, it begins to translate into true feelings of self-worth and real-world success. 'Change your thoughts and you change your world,' is one of Peale's famous sayings, along with advice such as, 'When you get up in the morning, you have two choices – either to be happy or to be unhappy. Just choose to be happy.'

So try it. When you get up in the morning, instead of looking in the mirror and telling yourself what a loser you are, instead try telling yourself that you're a winner and that you deserve success. If you're having a hard time, go to the one or two people who you know best, the ones you can really count on. Not all of us, but most of us, have such people in our lives. Tell them, 'I'm having a really hard time right now. Can you tell me a few things you like about me?' Write those things down and stick them on a mirror. And when you look in the mirror you'll be reminded of the positive things others see in you.

In addition to voicing positive words, acting out positive thoughts can have an impact too. Behavioural psychologists call this the 'fake-it-till-you-make-it' school. Act like a success, and you – along with the people around you – will start to believe that you *are* a success. Act like you're happy and you'll start to become happier.

Take smiling. Psychologists have long believed that people who smile more have more positive lives and, as a consequence, are happier, healthier and live longer. One study analysed photographs of baseball players from the 1950s. The study showed that those who smiled the most, versus players who were never smiling in their photos, lived an average of seven years longer.[1]

Now, maybe the baseball players who smiled were just happier to begin with. But here's the odd finding: if you make yourself smile, even if you don't mean it, and you keep at it, pretty soon you'll not only find yourself smiling more, you'll enjoy the associated health benefits as well. Smiling is a signal to the rest of your body that counteracts the effects of stress. It convinces your body that things are good, so actually releases good hormones and improves your mood – something that scientists have confirmed with brain scans.[2]

Smiles are also contagious, so people around you respond more positively. A whole positive, self-reinforcing loop gets started, just like the positive loop you start by saying encouraging things to yourself. So instead of buying the world a Coke, as the commercial says, give the world your best grin.

Respecting yourself means positive actions

Everyone on the planet knows the things they shouldn't be doing. Pick your poison: smoking cigarettes, drinking too much coffee, having too much wine, not eating enough fruit and veggies, eating too much steak, using too many recreational drugs . . . It's not like we don't know this stuff is bad for us.

Part of self-respect is about trying to be good to ourselves, and trying to do fewer of the bad things. And here's the positive spin: the more good things we do for ourselves, the better we feel, which leads to more positive actions.

I think a big reason that negativity drops away during a Reboot is because the action we are taking dramatically changes our opinion of ourselves. We're really doing something to change our lives. You go 10 days without your usual food, drinking only juice or consuming only fruits and veggies, which is most likely the first time you've done that in your life. When you achieve that, you feel great about yourself. You start to look at yourself in a different way, with a lot more confidence and a lot less negativity.

The same thing goes for other actions you take, be they getting enough exercise, or sleeping well, or even making sure that when it comes to community and intimacy you are spending time with positive people and those who support your mission.

When it comes to actions, the inverse is also true. It's seems wildly obvious, but just don't do things that make you hate yourself. The reason I don't drink alcohol any more (I haven't had a drink since I started my journey in 2007) is not because alcohol was detrimental to my health – though too much of it certainly is – but because there were too many mornings after a night out on the town when I regretted some of the things I said and did. I didn't like that person I became, so I felt depressed and hated myself the next day. Eventually I said, 'What's the point of this? I'm going out, having a few drinks and enjoying myself for three hours, then feeling terrible for 72 hours.' The mathematical formula of risk and reward, of gain and pain, didn't pay off. It was time to put the bottle away.

Being kind to yourself when 'pizza happens'

One of our medical advisers, Dr Carrie Diulus, talks about her family's eating philosophy in *Fat, Sick & Nearly Dead 2*. I suspect she might someday be famous for her observation that although they are a 'mostly plants' family, sometimes 'pizza happens'. I expect to see it as a bumper sticker any day now.

What the phrase means is that even for the best of us, for the most vigilantly healthy, slip-ups occur. The crucial thing is not whether we'll slip up – as humans, that's pretty much inevitable – but how we deal with it.

We're not talking about the evening you go out and have some treat that you've planned on giving yourself as a reward for good behaviour. We're talking about the accidental slide.

Here is something that happens to more people than you can possibly imagine. You start the night out at 7pm and say, 'I'm going to be really good tonight and have only vegetables,' or 'I'm going to pass on that spaghetti carbonara,' or 'I'm going to avoid any sugary desserts.' But by 9pm you've eaten 3,000 calories of absolute twaddle. You ask yourself, 'How the hell did this happen?' which quickly descends to, 'Why am I such a loser?'

Is this splurge of overeating a cry for help? Is it an act of mindless eating? Or is it just a crazy act of self-indulgence because things have been tough and stressful lately? Maybe it started out as an innocent, 'I'll just have this piece of candy' and it then spiralled out of control.

Guess what? It doesn't matter why you did it. What matters is how you react. The worst thing, and an Achilles' heel for all dieters, is to go down the rabbit hole of self-disgust, which then opens the door for a boatload of self-destructive behaviour. Since you were bad to eat that bowl of ice cream, you throw yourself under the bus by eating the whole tub.

This is a pivotal defining moment. If you find yourself in such a position – be it the moment after or the morning after – you need to pull the plug on self-hate right then and there.

'Pizza happens' means sometimes we eat more pizza than we planned to. It means we sometimes go farther than we should. Maybe we thought we could have a bowl of ice cream but had the whole carton instead. OK, let's focus on eating more veggies the next night and wait to have some more ice cream when you feel like you've really earned it. Give yourself leeway to go out of bounds, but don't use straying as an excuse to abandon your boundaries. Don't turn it into a slide. This is part of loving yourself – not being so hard on yourself, but being kind and forgiving, just as you would be to someone you loved.

I think that one of the reasons that very strict diets invariably fail is that they grant no leeway. Everything that is foolish and fun is taken away; you run a totally tight ship until, one day, everything explodes and comes crashing down.

The way I see it, it's much better to forgive yourself ahead of time – to plan for and be conscious of those times when you can reward yourself with a treat. That greatly changes the dynamic of 'breaking' your diet.

Before I did my first Reboot, one of my favourite go-to foods was a cheeseburger. After my Reboot I avoided meat for four years. I'm not sure if I was just not interested, or if I was seriously concerned that a single bite would send me over the edge. Three years ago I had a cheeseburger, very deliberately and planned out. Since then I've had a cheeseburger on rare occasions once every two months or so. They were homemade, and I enjoyed each and every one of those times. I never felt guilty because each time was a conscious decision and a reward for having been very conscientious about my nutrition.

But had the scenario been different – had I suddenly blurted out to the waitress, 'Bring me a cheeseburger,' when all along I was planning to order a spinach salad – that would have been a different story. So, rather like calling food good or bad, the context is everything. Demonizing the food itself gives food the power.

I choose instead to decide if and when I'm going to eat something that doesn't fit into a purely nutritious diet. I'll then choose something I'm really going to enjoy – like my favourite chocolate ice cream – rather than some random dessert that just happens to be within view at the time.

And in the end . . .

We've spent a lot of time talking about respecting yourself, and how important that is for you to have the power to live a healthy life, which is the only path to leading a happy life.

In some ways, we are talking about a moral compass and the knowledge we all have inside ourselves about doing the right thing. While it's not a script for a morality play, the reality is that if you do the right thing, you'll respect yourself for doing it. What's equally important is to not hate yourself or beat yourself up for making mistakes. That's not being morally bad, that's just being weak and human. That's where perspective comes in.

If you ask me what the secret to happiness is, I have to

go back to what the Jesuits taught me as a kid – that we are here to serve others. Personally, I think the secret to happiness is being useful, and the more useful you are, the happier you are. When you're useful, you're taking action, you're doing something, you're participating and you're contributing. In many ways, the idea of loving and respecting yourself is really played out by what you do for – and to – others. Yes, it's also what you do to and for yourself, but you can love and respect yourself by loving, respecting and helping others.

If you're lucky, and you work at it, you might have a lot of great moments where it all comes together. Just like when you experience the Reboot, it's about a combination of things coming together: it's the right nutrients hitting your system and the wrong ones being avoided; it's having good sleep, exercise and rest; it's three or four days of feeling good about yourself. All these things comes together to give us that beautiful day, inside and outside our minds, so that we see ourselves as worthwhile, positive and optimistic about what we're doing and what we've achieved. And I think that respecting yourself – the combination of honouring and caring for yourself – brings you confidence, happiness and love.

TIPS FOR BUILDING SELF-RESPECT

1 **Write a list** of 10 things that make you feel good about yourself – accomplishments, actions and attributes. Then write a list of 10 reasons why other people like you. Or ask one or two people you are close to to list some reasons they like you.

2 **Become sensitive to the negative inner voice** that says you are worthless for doing (or not doing) something. Whenever you are aware of it, just stop it and tell yourself instead that you're wonderful and you'll do better next time.

3 **Practise morning affirmations.** Write affirmative notes and put them on your bathroom mirror. And tell yourself every morning when you wake up that this is going to be the best day of your life, and that you can accomplish anything you want.

More than anything else, says Londoner Christopher Treloar, what keeps him from going back to his old eating habits is the inspirational voice inside his head.

'When I was at my biggest, the problem was that this inner voice was telling me you're big anyway, so eating more won't make that big a difference. That was the worst message I could hear.'

Since going on a 96-day Reboot in the spring of 2013 and losing 6 stone (84 pounds) – which he has kept off – he says there's a new voice. 'Now I've got my weight down, I want to keep going; I want to get even healthier. The voice I'm hearing now speaks in phrases from motivational speeches. So if there is a moment when I'm at my weakest, when I'm thinking I want to eat something I shouldn't, then I have that voice . . . It's the speech from *Rocky*, or even the voice from *Braveheart*, which has no particular significance for me, but is inspirational all the same. Sometimes it's Billy Bob Thornton in *Friday Night Lights* . . . I keep those voices in my head on a day-to-day basis, motivating myself to think healthy, to think positive and not ruin all the stuff I've already done that day for myself.'

For Christopher, an online content creator, the moment of truth came when he was watching an episode of *The Simpsons*, where Homer was trying to reach 21 stone (300 pounds) so he could be classified as morbidly obese. At the time, Christopher was 299 pounds. 'That is when it kind of hit home. I had become a fat Homer, basically.'

After trying Weight Watchers, which he says worked for about a month before 'the old habits crept back in', a friend sent him a link to watch *Fat, Sick & Nearly Dead*.

'I'll never forget the moment. I was lying in bed at the time. It was about 10.30 in the morning. I had only one son at the time [he now has two]. He was three and was off playing. I didn't even have the energy to play with him,' he says. 'I was fixated by the film. I saw a bit of myself in Joe.' Before it was half over, he had ordered a juicer from a local store. 'I started juicing that day.'

Since then he has become a regular runner, including taking part in the London Marathon. He calls that race his 'healthiversary', since it took place a year after he started juicing. 'This was no part of me whatsoever beforehand. But I've kind of caught this running bug.'

Christopher says he's had a weight problem all his life, beginning with overeating as a child. 'My mum, bless her, was a bit of a feeder. Our portion sizes were just obscene. It was only when I was juicing that I was able to sit back and [realize] how much we had on our plates.' He and his brother also developed the habit of 'tucking into the crisps [potato chips] and chocolate bars' after school each day.

He credits his girlfriend, a nurse, with making him aware of his food cravings and what they were doing to his health. 'The biggest challenge I've got is this food addiction. I denied it for years, but I'd be eating chocolate bars and crisps late at night and then hiding the wrappers.' She also went so far as to film him while he was sleeping, to show him how bad his sleep apnoea had become thanks to being overweight.

Today, one of his basic tools is simply to cut portions in half, augmented by lots of fresh juice. 'I was a guy who was eating two sandwiches for lunch, two chocolate bars and crisps. I've stripped that back to one sandwich and some fruit for lunch, and I keep juicing most days because then I'm getting all the good stuff into my body.'

Christopher says he still eats 'the odd chocolate bar here or there', but is now aware of his eating habits and adjusts accordingly. 'If there is a day when I go out and have a big meal with people, I'm always aware of what I've just done, and ways I can exercise and drink some juice and fight it off, rather than just keep going and piling it on like I've done before.'

He says he's motivated by having two young sons, who need him to be energetic – and he has never gotten over the energy he experienced during his first Reboot, when he says he felt like he was 'on top' of the Tower of London.

'The other thing that motivates me is to look at old photos. We've still got pictures of me around the house from when I was at my biggest. It's looking at those and thinking, "Here is a picture of me standing outside the stadium during the Olympics and I'm wearing a triple-X T-shirt." At no stage do I ever want to go back to being that guy again.'

CONCLUSION

By the time you read this book you will have seen – or at least have had the opportunity to see – *Fat, Sick & Nearly Dead 2*. You will have seen and met some of the people I did. People who changed their lives. People who changed their communities. People who had the courage to face their struggle with bad diet, bad health and bad habits, and do something about it.

One of our working titles for the movie was 'Life after Juice', but that wasn't quite right. It wasn't *after* but *alongside* juice. Even when people come down from the mountaintop of a Reboot and return to the world of eating, they don't want to give up their reborn love for a plant-rich diet and the power of fresh juice. They make it part of a new way of life; they take it along with them as they continue their personal journeys.

For me, the film was another chapter in my own learning curve, another step in my quest to understand what it takes to maintain a healthy lifestyle in a world that doesn't make it easy. As always, I consulted plenty of experts. But I learned even more from the people I met and talked to along the way. I've tried to put those ideas in this book, not so much as a plan, but as a toolkit of things that worked for them and for me. And they just might work for you – though that depends.

I was proud and humbled that my story and my little film played a role in inspiring their journeys. And 'inspire' is the right word. Because something else I've learned is that when it comes to making changes, not many of us like to be told what to do. We want to discover things for ourselves, or at least confirm them for ourselves. About the best thing you can do is to lead by example, and that is what I've tried to do – not to tell people what to do, but to show them what's possible, even for an ordinary guy like myself.

So what's my biggest takeaway from life after the Reboot? I will tell you a couple of things I'm now certain of, having seen many success stories, and some not so successful. One is that you can't do it alone. You need a community, whether it's family, friends, people in your town, or a group of folks you can talk to online. But whatever it is in your life that you want to change, there is a community out there waiting for you.

The other thing I'm pretty sure about is that, however you do it, the more fruit and vegetables you can get into your system, the better off you're going to be. So go ahead and make yourself a juice, or grab a salad, or whip up a smoothie. And give my best to Mother Nature. She's waiting to give her best to you.

Part III
RESOURCES

WEEKLY MENU PLANNER

Below is my typical week's menu. As you know by now, my diet is plant-based, which means that I try to get the majority of my calories from plants, but I do still have some animal products. I've provided alternatives to these for those who are vegetarian or vegan.

Key
V = vegan options
AF = anti-inflammatory additions
GF = gluten-free options

MEAL	MONDAY	TUESDAY	WEDNESDA*
BREAKFAST	*Delicious Detox Juice* (page 189)	*Vegetable Omelette* (page 197) **V:** replace eggs with tofu	*Morning Orang Juice* (page 19(**AF:** add turmeri
LUNCH	*Vegan Salad* (page 203)	Mixed greens or lettuce wrap with chicken, avocado, spinach & sprouts **V:** replace chicken with hummus	*Fiesta Quinoa Salad* (page 20
DINNER	*Asian-inspired Veggie Stir-fry* (page 212)	Grilled tuna & asparagus **V:** replace tuna with grilled aubergine (eggplant) or vegetable kebabs	*Courgette (Zucchini) 'Pasta Primavera* (page 210)
SNACK	*Super-easy Hummus* (page 217) with carrot & celery sticks	*Green Berry Smoothie* (page 195)	Apple slices & almond butter
TREAT		*Sweet Treat Smoothie* (page 194)	

THURSDAY	FRIDAY	SATURDAY	SUNDAY
et Potato cakes (page	*Spicy Veggie Scramble* (page 199)	*Wake-up Red Juice* (page 191) **AF:** add turmeric	Warmed pinhead (steel-cut) oats with flaxseed & berries **GF:** use gluten-free oats
eplace egg flaxseed '	**V:** replace eggs with tofu		
sic green d with *Lemon ken* (page), tomatoes & :ado	*Green Smoothie* (page 193)	Kale (Tuscan cabbage) salad with grilled prawns (shrimp)	*Vegan Spicy Parsnip Celeriac Soup* (page 201)
eplace chicken chickpeas (in d) or hummus vrap)		**V:** replace prawns (shrimp) with sunflower seeds, almonds, chia seeds	
an Spiced ls Over liflower 'Rice' e 208) add turmeric	*Salmon Patty* (page 213) **V:** replace salmon with Portobello Mushroom Wraps (page 214)	*Classic Greens with Lemon Chicken* (page 206) **V:** replace chicken with baked tofu	Cauliflower Crust Pizza (page 215)
en Smoothie e 193)	*Homemade Healthy Granola Bar* (page 219)	*Guacamole* (page 218) with carrots or daikon radish/ jicama sticks or wholegrain crackers	*Joe's Mean Green* (page 192) **AF:** add turmeric
g/2 oz dark :olate		100–175 g/4–6 oz ice cream	50 g/2 oz *Macadamia Date Balls* (page 221)

RECIPES

Please note the following general points, which apply to all the recipes.

- All the recipes use standard UK/US spoon measures: 1 teaspoon (tsp) = 5 ml; 1 tablespoon (tbsp) = 15 ml. Note that in Australia 1 tsp = 5 ml, but 1 tbsp = 20 ml, so take care when measuring. All spoonfuls should be level.

- A handful is equal to about 8 oz/250 ml/1 cup.

- All eggs and produce are medium in size, unless a recipe states otherwise.

- Wash all produce (preferably in a vinegar and water solution – see below) before juicing, blending or cooking it.

- Please note that the nutrition information for juices is just an estimate. The actual calories and nutritional content will vary based on the size of your produce and the efficiency of your juicer.

- If using canned foods, such as beans or tomatoes, some authorities (such as the US Food and Drug Administration) advise against cans where the inside is coated with Biphenol-A (BPA), an industrial chemical that can transfer into food. The same goes for plastic storage containers and bottles made with this chemical. Some research studies have linked BPA to breast cancer and diabetes, as well as to hyperactivity, aggression and depression in children.

Produce Wash

I usually wash all produce, including anything that will be peeled, with water. But if you are concerned about pesticides and/or food-borne bacteria, the following wash is a great natural disinfectant.

8 fl oz/250 ml/1 cup water
8 fl oz/250 ml/1 cup white vinegar
1 tbsp bicarbonate of soda (baking soda)
juice of ½ lemon

1 Mix the ingredients in a large bowl to allow for the vigorous chemical reaction between the vinegar and bicarb. When the reaction has stopped, pour the liquid into a spray bottle.
2 Spray your produce (you can scrub firm items), then rinse well.

Juices

Delicious Detox Juice

Makes 1 serving (16-20 oz/500-600 ml/2-2½ cups)

Nutrition per serving: 157 kCal; 655 kJ; 6 g protein; 52 g carbohydrates; 1 g fat; 0 g saturated fat; 3 g fibre; 26 g sugar; 145 mg sodium

1 celery stick
½ lemon, peeled
¼ head of red cabbage
3 carrots
1 orange, peeled
3 in/7.5 cm fresh turmeric root or ½ tsp ground turmeric

1 Prepare the ingredients, and cut to size for your juicer.
2 Feed everything, except the ground turmeric, through the juicer.
3 Pour the juice into a glass, stir in the ground turmeric (if using), and enjoy.

Morning Orange Juice

Makes 1 serving (16–20 oz/500–600 ml/2–2½ cups)

Nutrition per serving: 136 kCal; 568 kJ; 5 g protein; 45 g carbohydrates; 1 g fat; 0 g saturated fat; 5 g fibre; 27 g sugar; 133 mg sodium

  3 carrots

  2 oranges, peeled

  ½ lemon, peeled

  1 sweet red (bell) pepper (capsicum), deseeded

  1 in/2.5 cm piece of fresh root ginger

1 Prepare the ingredients, and cut to size for your juicer.

2 Feed everything through the juicer.

3 Pour the juice into a glass and enjoy.

Wake-up Red Juice

Makes 1 serving (16-20 oz/500-600 ml/2-2½ cups)

Nutrition per serving: 159 kCal; 666 kJ; 5 g protein; 54 g carbohydrates; 1 g fat; 0 g saturated fat; 4 g fibre; 25 g sugar; 229 mg sodium

- 3 carrots
- 1 apple, cored
- 1 beetroot (beet), peeled
- ½ lemon, peeled
- 4 Swiss chard leaves

1 Prepare the ingredients, and cut to size for your juicer.

2 Feed everything through the juicer.

3 Pour the juice into a glass and enjoy.

Joe's Mean Green

Makes 1 serving (16–20 oz/500–600 ml/2–2½ cups)

Nutrition per serving: 251 kCal; 1049 kJ; 6 g protein; 54 g carbohydrates; 1 g fat; 0 g saturated fat; 2 g fibre; 30 g sugar; 128 mg sodium

    8 kale (Tuscan cabbage) leaves
    1 cucumber
    4 celery sticks
    2 apples, cored
    ½ lemon, peeled
    1 in/2.5 cm piece of fresh root ginger

1 Prepare the ingredients, and cut to size for your juicer.

2 Feed everything through the juicer.

3 Pour the juice into a glass and enjoy.

Smoothies

Green Smoothie

Makes 2 servings (16-20 oz/500-600 ml/2-2½ cups)

Nutrition per serving: 189 kCal; 791 kJ; 4 g protein; 36 g carbohydrates; 5 g fat; 0 g saturated fat; 0 g fibre; 21 g sugar; 119 mg sodium

12 fl oz/350 ml/1½ cups almond milk

1 banana, peeled

½ cucumber

½ lime, peeled

¼ pineapple, peeled and cored

4 mint leaves

2 tbsp flaxseed

1 handful of ice (3-4 cubes)

1 Prepare the ingredients and place them in a blender.
2 Whiz on high speed for 45–60 seconds, then pour into a glass and enjoy.

Sweet Treat Smoothie

Makes 1 serving (16-20 oz/500-600 ml/2-2½ cups)

Nutrition per serving: 254 kCal; 1062 kJ; 4 g protein; 25 g carbohydrates; 15 g fat; 7 g saturated fat; 8 g fibre; 8 g sugar; 181 mg sodium

½ banana, peeled, then frozen

1 tsp vanilla extract

½ tbsp ground cinnamon

10 fl oz/280 ml/1¼ cup unsweetened almond milk

2 tbsp raw cacao nibs

1 handful of ice (3-4 cubes)

1 Prepare the ingredients and place them in a blender.

2 Whiz on high speed for 45-60 seconds, then pour into a glass and enjoy.

Green Berry Smoothie

Makes 1 serving (16-20 oz/500-600 ml/2-2½ cups)

Nutrition per serving: 82 kcal; 343 kJ; 2 g protein; 19 g carbohydrates; 1 g fat; 0 g saturated fat; 3 g fibre; 11 g sugar; 108 mg sodium

2 oz/50 g/½ cup fresh or frozen raspberries
2 oz/50 g/½ cup fresh or frozen strawberries
1 handful of spinach
½ lemon, peeled
3 mint leaves
6 fl oz/190ml/¾ cup coconut water
1 handful of ice (3-4 cubes)

1 Prepare the ingredients and place them in a blender.
2 Whiz on high speed for 45–60 seconds, then pour into a glass and enjoy.

Breakfasts

Vegetable Omelette

Makes 1 serving

Nutrition per serving: 399 kCal; 1669 kJ; 21 g protein; 19 g carbohydrates; 27 g fat; 4 g saturated fat; 7 g fibre; 6 g sugar; 303 mg sodium

1 tbsp olive oil

½ small onion, diced

1 egg plus 3 egg whites

1 garlic clove, crushed (minced)

8oz/225g/1 cup cherry tomatoes, halved

1 handful of spinach, chopped

¼ jalapeño chilli pepper, diced (optional)

¼ avocado

1 small handful of parsley, chopped

1 Heat the olive oil in a frying pan (skillet) set over a medium heat. Add the onion and sauté until golden.

2 Whisk the egg, egg whites and garlic together in a small bowl. Add the tomatoes, spinach and chilli.

3 Pour the egg mixture into the frying pan (skillet) and cook for 3–4 minutes, until the underside is lightly browned and the surface is beginning to firm up. Fold in half and continue to cook for another 2 minutes, until the centre is firm.

4 Garnish with the avocado and parsley. Serve immediately.

Sweet Potato Pancakes

Makes 4 servings

Nutrition per serving: 90 kCal; 380 kJ; 3 g protein; 184 g carbohydrates; 1 g fat; 1 g saturated fat; 3 g fibre; 6 g sugar; 51 mg sodium

2 eggs or 4 egg whites (for vegans, replace whole eggs with 2 tbsp ground flaxseed mixed with 6 tbsp water and allow to gel before using – takes about 10 minutes)

1 sweet potato, baked

1 banana, peeled

2 tbsp coconut flour

½ tsp ground cinnamon

1 tbsp coconut oil

ground nutmeg (optional)

sea salt, to taste

1 Whisk the eggs in a bowl.

2 Mash the sweet potato and banana together in a separate bowl. Add the eggs, coconut flour, cinnamon, ginger and salt.

3 Heat the coconut oil in a frying pan (skillet) over a medium heat.

4 Spoon some batter into the pan, spreading it smooth and flat with the back of the spoon. Cook each side until brown, about 5 minutes.

5 Repeat with remaining batter to make 3 more pancakes.

6 Serve with a dash of nutmeg if you wish, or top with apple sauce.

Spicy Veggie Scramble

Makes 1 serving

Nutrition per serving: 312 kCal; 1305 kJ; 16 g protein; 16 g carbohydrates; 21 g fat; 8 g saturated fat; 7 g fibre; 5 g sugar; 195 mg sodium

   2 eggs
   1 garlic clove, crushed (minced)
   1 tomato, chopped
   1 handful of spinach, chopped
   ¼ jalapeño chilli pepper, diced (optional)
   1 tsp coconut oil
   ¼ avocado, cubed
   1 small handful of coriander (cilantro), chopped

1 Whisk the eggs and garlic together in a small bowl. Add the tomato, spinach and chilli.

2 Heat the coconut oil in a frying pan (skillet) over a medium heat.

3 Pour in the egg mixture and cook, stirring, until it is cooked through (about 3 minutes).

4 Garnish with the avocado and coriander. Serve immediately.

Main Dishes

Vegan Spicy Parsnip Celeriac Soup

Makes 3 servings

Nutrition per serving: 297 kCal; 1242 kJ; 5 g protein; 57 g carbohydrates; 6 g fat; 1 g saturated fat; 12 g fibre; 13 g sugar; 277 mg sodium

1 tbsp olive oil

1 small onion, diced

1 leek, white and pale green parts only, thinly sliced

4 garlic cloves, crushed (minced)

1¼ lb/550 g/3 cups parsnips, peeled and chopped

1 small head of celeriac, peeled and cubed

generous pinch of crushed black pepper

¼ tsp cayenne pepper

¼ tsp ground turmeric

12 fl oz/350 ml/1½ cups low-sodium vegetable stock

12 fl oz/350 ml/1½ cups water

6 fl oz /175 ml/¾ cup unsweetened almond milk

3 spring onions (scallions), green ends only, chopped, for garnish

1 Place the olive oil in a large saucepan over a medium heat.

2 Add the onion and cook for 2 minutes.

3 Add the leek and garlic and cook for another 3 minutes.

4 Add the parsnips, celeriac, black pepper, cayenne and turmeric. Cook for 3 minutes.

5 Add the stock and water and bring to the boil. Cover and simmer until the vegetables are very soft, about 30 minutes. Set aside to cool slightly.

6 Purée the soup, then stir in the almond milk.

7 Serve in individual bowls, garnished with the spring onions.

Vegan Salad

Makes 3–4 servings

Nutrition per serving: 289 kCal; 1212 kJ; 10 g protein; 18 g carbohydrates; 21 g fat; 2 g saturated fat; 1 g fibre; 5 g sugar; 127 mg sodium

5 kale (Tuscan cabbage) leaves, chopped

¼ head of red cabbage, chopped

½ small red onion, chopped

2 tbsp chia seeds

1¼ oz/35 g/¼ cup sunflower seeds

2¼ oz/60 g/¼ cup raw walnuts

For the dressing

1 tsp Dijon mustard

2 tsp finely grated lemon zest

3 tbsp fresh lemon juice

6 tbsp extra virgin olive oil

sea salt and freshly ground pepper, to taste

1 Place all the salad ingredients in a large bowl.

2 Combine all the dressing ingredients in a small bowl and whisk together.

3 Pour the dressing over the salad and toss until evenly coated. Allow to marinate for 1 hour, if desired, then serve.

Fiesta Quinoa Salad

Makes 2 servings

Nutrition per serving: 318 kCal; 1330 kJ; 9 g protein; 43 g carbohydrates; 12 g fat; 1 g saturated fat; 12 g fibre; 4 g sugar; 27 mg sodium

9 oz/250 g/1 cup quinoa, cooked according to packet directions

4½ oz/120 g/½ cup canned low-sodium black beans (BPA-free), rinsed and drained

7 cos (romaine) lettuce leaves, chopped

½ sweet red (bell) pepper (capsicum), sliced

¼ red onion, sliced

1 plum tomato, sliced

¼ avocado, cubed

2 tbsp chopped fresh coriander (cilantro)

To serve

1 lime, halved

1 tbsp olive oil

dash of hot chilli sauce (optional)

1 Layer the salad ingredients in a bowl in the order listed above.

2 Just before serving, squeeze some lime juice over the salad, then sprinkle with the olive oil and hot chilli sauce (if using).

Variation

If you'd like to serve the salad hot, do as follows. While the quinoa is cooking, sauté the peppers and onions in olive oil until soft, about 3 minutes. Add the tomatoes and sauté for

1 minute, then add the black beans and heat through (about 3 minutes). Serve over the warm quinoa and lettuce. Top with the avocado, a squeeze of lime juice and the olive oil, adding the hot chilli sauce if you wish.

Classic Greens with Lemon Chicken

Makes 1 serving

Nutrition per serving: 443 kCal; 2138 kJ; 34 g protein; 15 g carbohydrates; 28 g fat; 5 g saturated fat; 5 g fibre; 7 g sugar; 947 mg sodium

1 boneless chicken breast

4 tsp olive oil

8 asparagus spears

2 large handfuls of mixed greens

1 tomato, chopped

1 tbsp chopped walnuts

sea salt and freshly ground pepper

For the dressing

juice of 1 lemon

1 tbsp balsamic vinegar

1 tsp Dijon mustard

1 tbsp olive oil

1 Preheat the oven to 375°F/190°C/gas 5. Line 2 baking sheets with foil.

2 Rub both sides of the chicken breast with half the olive oil, then sprinkle with salt and pepper. Place on a prepared baking sheet and roast for 45 minutes, or until the internal temperature reaches 165°F/74°C. Set aside to cool before chopping.

3 Snap off and discard the woody ends of the asparagus. Place the spears on a prepared baking sheet, drizzle with the remaining oil and toss to coat. Roast in a single layer for about 15 minutes, until tender.

4 Meanwhile, make the dressing. Whisk the lemon juice,

vinegar and mustard together in a small bowl. While still whisking, add the olive oil to create emulsion.

5 Combine the greens, tomato, asparagus and chopped chicken in a large bowl. Add the dressing and toss to coat. Sprinkle with the walnuts.

Indian Spiced Lentils over Cauliflower 'Rice'

Makes 4 servings

Nutrition per serving: 341 kCal; 1426 kJ; 12 g protein; 49 g carbohydrates; 11g fat; 5 g saturated fat; 16 g fibre; 19 g sugar; 179 mg sodium

11 oz/300 g/1½ cups brown lentils

1 tbsp olive oil

1 large onion, chopped

3 garlic cloves, crushed (minced)

2 tsp ground cumin

2 tsp ground coriander

2 tsp ground paprika

1 tsp chopped jalapeño chilli pepper, optional

2 sweet red (bell) peppers (capsicums), chopped

2 carrots, diced

1 celery stick, chopped

16 fl oz/475 ml/2 cups vegetable stock

16 fl oz/475 ml/2 cups water

2 lb/900 g/4 cups chopped tomatoes

freshly ground pepper, to taste

For the cauliflower 'rice'

½ head of cauliflower

1 tbsp coconut oil

8 fl oz/250 ml/1 cup coconut milk

¼ tsp black pepper

¼ tsp ground turmeric

To garnish

1 small handful of fresh coriander (cilantro), chopped

1 small handful of fresh parsley, chopped

1 Rinse the lentils under cold water.

2 Place the olive oil in a large flameproof casserole dish (Dutch oven) over a medium heat. Add the onion and garlic and cook until soft, about 3 minutes. Add the ground spices and chilli pepper and cook until fragrant, about 3 minutes.

3 Add the red peppers, carrots and celery and continue to cook, stirring occasionally, for a few minutes. Add the lentils, stock, water, tomatoes and pepper and cook, covered, over a low heat for 45 minutes, or until the lentils are tender.

4 Meanwhile, cut cauliflower into large florets. Whiz in a food processor (about 4 at a time) until the texture is 'rice-like'. Transfer to a bowl.

5 Heat the coconut oil in a large frying pan (skillet) over a medium-high heat. Add the whizzed cauliflower and cook 3 minutes, stirring occasionally.

6 Add the coconut milk, pepper and turmeric, and continue to cook, stirring occasionally, for 3 more minutes.

7 Place the cauliflower in a serving bowl and spoon the lentil mixture over the top. Garnish with chopped parsley and coriander.

Courgette (Zucchini) 'Pasta' Primavera

Makes 4 servings

Nutrition per serving: 227 kCal; 949 kJ; 4 g protein; 21 g carbohydrates; 14 g fat; 2 g saturated fat; 6g fibre; 11 g sugar; 120 mg sodium

4 courgettes (zucchini)

2 tbsp olive oil

For the sauce

2 tbsp olive oil

1 onion, chopped

4 garlic cloves, chopped

1 tbsp ground cumin

3 carrots, peeled and chopped

1 handful of spinach

1 bunch of asparagus, chopped

5 oz/150 g/1 cup cherry tomatoes, halved

1 handful of fresh parsley, chopped

1 tbsp dried oregano, crushed

1 tbsp dried thyme, crushed

10 tomatoes, cored and chopped

sea salt and freshly ground pepper, to taste

1 First make the sauce. Place the olive oil in a flameproof casserole dish (Dutch oven) over a medium heat. Add the onion and garlic and cook until soft, about 3 minutes.

2 Add the cumin along with some salt and pepper and cook until fragrant, about 3 minutes.

3 Add the remaining vegetables and the herbs. Stir well, then add the tomatoes and cook, covered, for about 20 minutes.

4 While the sauce is cooking, use a spiralizer to cut the courgettes into long ribbons, placing a bowl underneath to catch them. Cut into the length that you prefer.

5 Heat the olive oil in a large frying pan (skillet) over a medium-low heat. Add the 'noodles' and cook until soft, about 5 minutes. (You can eat them uncooked if you wish.)

6 Serve the primavera sauce over the noodles.

Note: A spiralizer is a tool that is used to make long ribbons from vegetables. You can pick one up at a cooking store. If you don't own a spiralizer, you can slice the zucchini in a food processor or with a mandoline, or use a sharp knife to make thin strips.

Asian-inspired Veggie Stir-fry

Makes 2 servings

Nutrition per serving: 340 kCal; 1422 kJ; 9 g protein; 31 g carbohydrates; 22 g fat; 3 g saturated fat; 7 g fibre; 11 g sugar; 590 mg sodium

1 tbsp olive oil
1 onion, finely chopped
1 garlic clove, crushed (minced)
1 tbsp water
4 oz/100g/1 cup broccoli florets, chopped
1 sweet red (bell) pepper (capsicum), chopped
1 tbsp grated fresh root ginger
2 carrots, cut into matchsticks
¼ head of cabbage, thinly sliced
1 tbsp tamari (gluten-free)
1 tbsp dried chilli (red pepper) flakes
1 oz/25 g/¼ cup cashew nuts
1 tbsp sesame oil

1 Heat the olive oil in a large frying pan (skillet) or wok over a medium heat. Add the onion and garlic and cook until soft, about 3 minutes. Add the water, broccoli, bell pepper and ginger and cook for 2 minutes. Add the carrots and cabbage, cook for another 2 minutes.

2 Combine the tamari and crushed chilli pepper in a small bowl. Add to the pan along with the cashews and stir-fry for 5 minutes, until the vegetables start to soften.

3 Drizzle the sesame oil over the vegetables and serve alone, or over quinoa.

Salmon Patty

Makes 1 serving

Nutrition per serving: 371 kCal; 1552 kJ; 37 g protein; 7 g carbohydrates; 19g fat; 3 g saturated fat; 2 g fibre; 1 g sugar; 548 mg sodium

6 oz/175 g salmon, cooked

2 egg whites (for vegans replace with 1 tbsp ground flaxseed mixed with 3 tbsp water and allow to gel before using – takes about 10 minutes)

½ tbsp lemon juice

1 tbsp Dijon mustard

1 tbsp coconut flour

1 tsp fresh dill, chopped

1 tbsp olive oil

salt and freshly ground pepper, to taste

1 Shred the salmon in a small bowl with a fork. Add all the remaining ingredients, except the oil, and mash to combine.

2 Form the mixture into a patty and cook in the olive oil over a medium-high heat for 3–4 minutes on each side, until lightly golden brown.

3 Serve with a wholegrain bun or lettuce wrap, or over a bed of salad greens.

Portobello Mushroom Wraps

Makes 4 servings

Nutrition per serving: 168 kCal; 702 kJ; 4 g protein; 12 g carbohydrates; 10 g fat; 1.5 g saturated fat; 3 g fibre; 5 g sugar; 250 mg sodium

4 large Portobello mushroom caps

3 tbsp olive oil

2 fl oz/50 ml/¼ cup balsamic vinegar

1 clove garlic, crushed (minced)

1 tsp dried basil

1 tsp dried oregano

4 large lettuce leaves

sea salt and freshly ground pepper, to taste

1 Place the mushroom caps, domed-side up, in a dish.

2 Put 2 tablespoons of the olive oil in a small bowl, add the vinegar, garlic, herbs and seasoning and whisk together. Pour over the mushroom caps and set aside to marinate for 15 minutes.

3 Heat the remaining tablespoon of oil in a frying pan (skillet) over a medium heat. Reduce the heat to low, then add the mushroom caps. Cover and cook for about 5 minutes on each side, until tender, brushing now and then with the leftover marinade.

4 Wrap the mushrooms in the lettuce leaves or serve on a bed of mixed salad greens and serve straight away.

Cauliflower Crust Pizzas

Makes about 6 servings

Nutrition per serving: 278 kCal; 870 kJ; 28 g protein; 29 g carbohydrates; 7 g fat; 2 g saturated fat; 10 g fibre; 12 g sugar; 356 mg sodium

1 head of cauliflower

1 egg (for vegans replace with 1 tbsp ground flaxseed mixed with 3 tbsp water and allow to gel before using)

1 vegan egg (3 tbsp flaxseed, 6 tbsp water)

2 oz/50g/½ cup coconut flour

2½ fl oz/65 ml/⅓ cup water

2 tbsp nutritional yeast (optional)

salt and freshly ground pepper

For the toppings

1 tbsp olive oil

1 onion, chopped

2 garlic gloves, crushed (minced)

4 carrots, chopped

½ tbsp dried thyme

½ tbsp dried sage

½ tbsp dried basil

16 fl oz/475 ml/2 cups organic, sodium-free tomato passata (sauce)

8 kale (Tuscan cabbage) leaves, chopped

4¼ oz/110g/¾ cup cherry tomatoes, halved

1 lb/450 g organic minced (ground) turkey, cooked (optional)

1 Preheat the oven to 425°F/220°C/gas 7. Line two 26 cm/10 inch pizza pans with baking parchment.

2 Make the vegan egg. Mix flaxseed and water together in a small bowl. Leave for 10 minutes to gel and begin to set.

3 Cut the cauliflower into large florets. Place in a food processor (about 4 at a time) and whiz until they have a 'rice-like' texture. Transfer to a bowl.

4 Add the vegan egg, egg, coconut flour, water, yeast (if using) and mix well.

5 Divide the mixture equally between the prepared pans and flatten using your hands or another piece of baking parchment (the base should be quite thin – about 10 mm/½ inch – or it will become wet). Bake for 10–15 minutes, or until lightly browned.

6 Meanwhile, heat the olive oil in a frying pan (skillet) over a medium heat. Add the onion and garlic and cook until soft, about 3 minutes. Add the carrots, thyme, sage and basil and cook until the carrots are soft, about 5 minutes.

7 Spread the passata evenly over the pizza bases. Arrange the sautéed vegetables, tomatoes and turkey meat over the top.

8 Reduce the oven temperature to 400°F/200°C/gas 6 and return the pizzas to the oven. Cook for about 20 minutes, or until the edges are brown and the crust is no longer doughy.

9 Add some kale to each pizza and bake for another 3–5 minutes. Allow to cool slightly, then serve.

Snacks and Treats

Super-easy Hummus

Makes 8 servings

Nutrition per serving: 145 kCal; 606 kJ; 4 g protein; 13 g carbohydrates; 8 g fat; 1 g saturated fat; 1 g fibre; 0 g sugar; 181 mg sodium

4 tbsp tahini

2¼ fl oz/60 ml/¼ cup fresh lemon juice (about 1 large lemon)

2 tbsp olive oil, plus more for serving

1 large garlic clove, crushed (minced)

pinch of ground cumin

1 x 14 oz/400 g can low-sodium chickpeas (garbanzo beans), rinsed and drained

2–3 tbsp water (optional)

sea salt, to taste

dash of ground paprika, to serve

1 Place the tahini and lemon juice in a food processor or blender and whiz for 1 minute.

2 Add the oil, garlic, cumin and salt and blend for another minute.

3 Add the chickpeas and whiz until thick and smooth. (You might need to add the water to get the desired consistency.)

4 Place in serving bowl, drizzle with a little extra olive oil and sprinkle with paprika.

Guacamole

Makes 8 servings

Nutrition per serving: 82 kCal; 343 kJ; 1 g protein; 4 g carbohydrates; 7 g fat; 1 g saturated fat; 3 g fibre; 1 g sugar; 125 mg sodium

2 avocados, stones removed

2 tbsp lime juice

generous pinch of freshly ground pepper

generous pinch of chipotle chilli powder

sea salt, to taste

1 garlic clove, crushed (minced)

1 Scoop the avocado flesh into a bowl or food processor. Add all the remaining ingredients, then mash or process until smooth.

Homemade Healthy Granola Bar

Makes 12 bars

Nutrition per serving: 159 kCal; 667kJ; 3 g protein; 15 g carbohydrates; 10 g fat; 5 g saturated fat; 3 g fibre; 10 g sugar; 6 mg sodium

3 fl oz/85 ml/⅓ cup pure maple syrup

1 tbsp macadamia butter

2 tbsp coconut flour

1½ oz/40 g/¼ cup chopped dates (about 4 dates)

1½ oz/40 g/¼ cup chopped dried cranberries (sulphite-free)

10 oz/275 g/1 cup chopped mixed nuts (almonds, pecans, Brazils, cashews)

3 oz/75 g/⅓ cup chopped pumpkin seeds

7 oz/200 g/1 cup coconut flakes

pinch of Himalayan salt or sea salt

1 Preheat the oven to 300°F/150°C/gas 2. Line an 8 x 8 in (20 x 20 cm) shallow baking tin (pan) with baking parchment.

2 Pour the maple syrup into a bowl, add the macadamia butter, coconut flour and salt and mix until well combined.

3 Add the chopped fruit, nuts, seeds and coconut flakes and mix thoroughly, using your hands.

4 Press the mixture firmly and evenly into the prepared tin. Bake for 20 minutes, then set aside to cool. You can (if you wish) place the mixture in the freezer for 1 hour or more to firm up further.

5 Once firm, use a sharp knife to cut into 12 bars. These can be stored in the fridge or freezer in an airtight container.

Variations

- Use any type of nut desired, in combination or alone.

- Omit the nuts and use a selection of seeds (pumpkin, sunflower seeds, sesame).

- Replace the dates with dried figs, raisins or sultanas.

- Use whatever dried fruit you like instead of cranberries – perhaps blueberries, figs, cherries or apricots.

- Try a different type of nut butter (almond, Brazil nut, cashew). Those who have a nut allergy could use sunflower butter.

- Replace the maple syrup with honey or brown rice syrup (malt syrup).

Note: Always chop nuts, seeds and dried fruit before measuring the amount needed.

Macadamia Date Balls

Makes 12 balls

Nutrition per serving: 120 kCal; 502 kJ; 1 g protein; 11 g carbohydrates; 9 g fat; 1.5 g saturated fat; 2 g fibre; 8 g sugar; 5 mg sodium

7 oz/200 g/1 cup macadamia nuts

5 fresh dates

5 dried figs

½ tsp vanilla extract

1 tsp cinnamon

2 tbsp coconut flour

pinch of Himalayan or sea salt

1 Place all the ingredients in a food processor or blender and whiz until ground and well combined.

2 Take teaspoonfuls of the mixture and roll into balls.

3 Store in an airtight container in the fridge.

Variations

- Replace the macadamias with any type of nut.
- For a nut-free option, use sesame seeds, pumpkin seeds or sunflower seeds.
- Replace the dates and figs with any dried fruit.

Exercise Planner

When it comes to the exercise part of the healthy living equation, I've learned that the 'best' exercise is whatever exercise someone *can* and *will* actually *do*, and will keep doing regularly! Whether that's walking, swimming, lifting weights, gardening or running around after young kids all day long – whatever gets someone out of the chair and moving around, it's all good.

What I've also learned is that we are all starting from very different places. We all need to respect our bodies, to appreciate them for what they can do today, and to look after them for the future. If you are new to exercise, it can be easy to start out too aggressively and at too high an intensity, thinking that this will get better or quicker results. In fact, that approach is counter-productive; research shows it usually leads to burn-out or even injury. Like so many healthy changes, the key to adopting an effective exercise programme is to develop habits that stick.

Reboot with Joe Cardio and Strength Workouts

To avoid the pitfalls of an aggressive start, if you are new to exercise or starting again after a break, you can find sample cardio and strength-training workouts at www.rebootwithjoe.com/fitness/workouts/

These workouts are based on simple principles that have been developed to assist everyone in our Reboot community to improve their health and well-being, whether on a Reboot or simply working towards a healthy lifestyle. We include both cardio and strength-training workouts with low-intensity and high-intensity options. Each workout comes with a detailed video that thoroughly explains the workout and each move to ensure correct form and alignment. Simply choose one cardio plan and one strength-training plan that best suit your fitness level and goals.

Cardio

1 Reboot walking workout: low intensity

The perfect way to get started. We provide you with a basic

programme that includes guidelines focusing on things such as how to warm up properly, how to know if you are walking fast enough, how much energy you should exert, and much more. Before you know it, our walking workout will have you off and running in no time!

2 Reboot jogging workout: high intensity

This is an interval training-based programme designed to take your fitness to the next level. We provide you with a detailed workout, together with information on factors such as proper jogging technique, how to balance the intensity of your training, and what juices you should consume for the most energy.

Strength training

1 Reboot movement workout: low intensity

This workout consists of five full-body exercises that have been specifically designed for our Reboot community. On this programme you'll rebalance your posture, alleviate aches and pains, and give yourself the confidence to take on more strenuous physical activities. Each exercise can be completed individually, together in a fun workout sequence, or added to your current fitness programme.

2 Reboot training workout: high intensity

This workout consists of five body-weight resistance-training exercises. It is a higher-intensity programme designed for those who have completed the Reboot movement workout and are looking for that next challenge. Shape and tone your body in a matter of weeks.

Joe's own weekly exercise programme

I've always found it easiest to focus on the cardio and strength aspects of an exercise routine – perhaps because of my rugby-playing youth. This year I've shifted that focus slightly. Strength training and cardio are still both very important to me, but I've also been including more yoga in my exercise routine, and I am working on building a meditation practice.

Below is my current weekly exercise plan. I'm not always able to follow it exactly because travel and other commitments sometimes get in the way. But I find that if I do achieve this level of exercise in a week, I feel pretty great.

SAMPLE MOVEMENT WEEK			
	Mon	Tues	Wed
Daily Meditation (depending on time available, 2-10 minutes of breathing, ei			
Yoga & Stretching (30-60 mins)	✓		✓
Core & Stretching (15-45 mins)		✓	
Strength Training	✓		✓
Cardio (Bike/Walk/Jog) 60 mins moderate intensity **OR** 30 mins higher intensity		✓	

Thurs	Fri	Sat	Sun
after waking or before going to bed)			
	✓	Rest day	
✓		Rest day	✓
	✓	Rest day	
✓		Rest day	Hike/Bike Outdoor Activity – something fun! 30-120 mins

Further Information

If you are interested in juicing and Rebooting, please check out www.rebootwithjoe.com. There you can also find out where to watch the movie that started it all, and that movie's sequel. My books are also excellent resources.

Documentary: *Fat, Sick & Nearly Dead* (2010)

Documentary: *Fat, Sick & Nearly Dead 2* (2014)

Joe Cross, *The Reboot with Joe Juice Diet* (Hodder & Stoughton, London; Greenleaf Book Group, Austin, TX, 2014)

Joe Cross, *The Reboot with Joe Juice Diet Recipe Book: Over 100 Recipes Inspired by the Film 'Fat, Sick & Nearly Dead'* (Hodder & Stoughton, London; Greenleaf Book Group, Austin, TX, 2014)

Further reading

If you're interested in further understanding your relationship with food and how to establish and maintain a healthy lifestyle, check out the following books, which have inspired me:

Joel Fuhrman, *The End of Dieting* (Hay House, London, 2014; HarperOne; New York, 2014)

Dr Fuhrman explains the key principles of the science of health, nutrition and weight loss. This book will give you a simple and effective strategy to achieve – and maintain – an optimal weight without dieting for the rest of your life.

Mark Hyman, *The Blood Sugar Solution: The Bestselling Programme for Preventing Diabetes, Losing Weight and Feeling Great* (Hodder & Stoughton, London, 2012; Little, Brown, New York, 2012)
Dr Hyman describes the seven keys to achieving wellness – nutrition, hormones, inflammation, digestion, detoxification, energy metabolism and a calm mind.

Michael Moss, *Salt Sugar Fat: How the Food Giants Hooked Us* (Random House, New York and London, 2013)
An eye-opening account of why breaking food addiction is so difficult for many of us.

Dean Ornish, *The Spectrum: A Scientifically Proven Program to Feel Better, Live Longer, Lose Weight, and Gain Health* (Ballantine Books, New York, 2008)
Dr Ornish's empowering new programme that enables you to customize a healthy way of eating and living based on your own desires, needs and genetic predispositions.

Michael Pollan, *In Defence of Food* (Penguin Books, London, 2009)
Michael is famous for having recommended a few years ago that we 'Eat Food. Not too much. Mostly plants.'

Brian Wansink, *Slim by Design: Mindless Eating Solutions for Everyday Life* (William Morrow, New York, 2014)

Professor Wansink's groundbreaking solutions for designing our most common spaces – schools, restaurants, grocery stores and home kitchens, among others – in order to make positive changes in how we approach and manage our diets.

Websites

The following links offer a variety of help and ideas.

Change4Life – www.nhs.uk/change4life
A government-sponsored website that offers lots of useful information about becoming happier and healthier.

Deepak Chopra – www.deepakchopra.com
Meditation resources, including many programmes and a free app.

Environmental Working Group's Food Scores – www.ewg.org/foodscores
This online database rates over 80,000 processed food items based on nutrition, ingredients and processing. So if you find yourself consuming processed food, consult this site for the best brands to select.

Get Some Headspace – www.headspace.com
Offers free 10-minute meditation programmes, including a free app.

Notes

Part I

The Journey Continues

1 'Preventable illness makes up approximately 70 per cent of the burden of illness and the associated costs. Well-developed national statistics, such as those outlined in *Healthy People 2000, Health U.S. 1991* and elsewhere, document this central fact clearly.' James F. Fries et al and the Health Project Consortium, 'Reducing Health Care Costs by Reducing the Need and Demand for Medical Services', *New England Journal of Medicine*, 329, 29 July 1993, pp.321–5.

Part II

1 Change Your Relationship with Food (Don't Abuse Food)

1 Brian Wansink, *Mindless Eating* (Bantam Books, New York, 2010), pp.140.
2 Wansink, op. cit., pp.16–18.
3 Michael Pollan, *The Botany of Desire* (Random House, New York, 2001), p.220.
4 Erik R. Trinidad, *Roadkill Café*, video from *Brain Games*, National Geographic Channel, broadcast August 2014 (www. youtube.com/watch?v=s4FRh2Crp_Q&feature=youtu.be).
5 Wansink, op. cit., pp.20–3.

6 Luigi Cornaro, *How to Live One Hundred Years*, first edition, 1566 (Kessinger Publishing LLC, Whitefish, MT, 2005); also www.drbass.com/cornaro.html, accessed 28 October 2014.

2 Change Your Diet (Eat the Right Stuff)

1 'Western Pattern Diet', Wikipedia, http://en.wikipedia.org/wiki/Western_pattern_diet, accessed 28 October 2014.

2 "CDC – Chronic Disease – Overview", Centers for Disease Control and Prevention, http://www.cdc.gov/ chronicdisease/overview/

3 Andrew J. Cooper et al., 'A Prospective Study of the Association Between Quantity and Variety of Fruit and Vegetable Intake and Incident Type 2 Diabetes', *Diabetes Care*, journal of the American Diabetes Association, 37(4), 4 April 2012.

4 Dariush Mozaffarian et al., 'Global Sodium Consumption and Death from Cardiovascular Causes', *New England Journal of Medicine*, 371, pp.624–34, 14 August 2014.

5 Samuel Soret et al., 'Climate change mitigation and health effects of varied dietary patterns in real-life settings throughout North America', *American Journal of Clinical Nutrition*, July 2014.

6 Tamlin S. Conner et al., 'On carrots and curiosity: Eating fruit and vegetables is associated with greater flourishing in daily life', *British Journal of Health Psychology*, first published online 30 July 2014.

7 Oyiniola Oyebode et al., 'Fruit and vegetable consumption and all-cause, cancer and CVD mortality: analysis of Health Survey for England data', *Journal of Epidemiology and Community Health*, 14 March 2014.

8 'List of countries by life expectancy', Wikipedia, http://en.wikipedia.org/wiki/List_of_countries_by_life_expectancy, accessed 28 October 2014.

9 S. Miyagi et al., 'Longevity and diet in Okinawa, Japan: the past, present and future', *Asia Pacific Journal of Public Health*, 2003, 5(S3–9).

10 Jonathan Foley, 'A Five Step Plan to Feed the World', *National Geographic*, May 2014, p.45.

3 Change Your Habits About Food (Find a New Groove)

1 David J. Linden, *The Compass of Pleasure* (Penguin Group, New York, 2011), pp.161–4.

2 David T. Neal et al., 'Habits – A Repeat Performance', *Current Directions in Psychological Science*, 2006, 15(4), pp.198–202.

3 Brian Wansink, *Mindless Eating* (Bantam Books, New York, 2010), pp.107–9.

4 Neal, op. cit., pp.198–202.

5 Wansink, op. cit., pp.78–80.

6 Stanley Schachter and Judith Rodin, *Obese Humans and Rats* (New York: John Wiley & Sons, 1974). 111–129

4 Embrace Community (Get a Little Help From Your Friends)

1 'Family Facts and Figures: Australian Households', Australian Institute of Family Studies (www.aifs.gov.au/institute/info/charts/households/#hprojected), accessed 28 October 2014.

2 'America's Families and Living Arrangements: 2012', US Census Bureau (www.census.gov/prod/2013pubs/p20–570.pdf), accessed 28 October 2014.

3 'Fifty years of families in Canada: 1961 to 2011', Statistics Canada (www.12.statcan.gc.ca/census–recensement/2011/as–sa/98–312–x/98–312–x2011003_1–eng.cfm), accessed 28 October 2014.

4 'Statistical Bulletin: Families and Households, 2012', Office for National Statistics (www.ons.gov.uk/ons/rel/family–

demography/families–and–households/2012/stb–families–households.html), accessed 28 October 2014.

5 J.D. Latner et al., 'Effective long-term treatment of obesity: a continuing care model', *International Journal of Obesity*, July 2000, 24(7), pp.893–8.

6 Dan Buettner, *The Blue Zones* (National Geographic Society, Washington DC, 2012), pp.89–91.

7 'Average Briton only has three true friends', *Daily Mail* (www.dailymail.co.uk/news/article–1266182/Average–Briton–THREE–true–friends–19–mates.html), accessed 28 October 2014.

8 'Close Friends Less Common Today, Study Finds', *Live Science* (www.livescience.com/16879–close–friends–decrease–today.html), accessed 28 October 2014.

9 Buettner, op. cit., pp.253–4.

10 'Our Friends' Weight Influences Our Weight Gain and Loss', *Scientific American* podcast (www.scientificamerican.com/podcast/episode/our–friends–weight–influences–our–w–12–07–15), 15 July 2012.

5 Maintain the Machine (Follow the Upkeep Manual)

1 J. Carson Smith et al., 'Physical activity reduces hippocampal atrophy in elders at genetic risk for Alzheimer's disease', *Frontiers in Aging Neuroscience*, 23 April 2014.

2 J.C. Smith et al., 'Interactive effects of physical activity and APOE-ε4 on BOLD semantic memory activation in healthy elders', *Neuroimage*, January 2011, 54(1), pp.635–44.

3 'Even More Reasons to Get a Move On', *New York Times* (www.nytimes.com/2010/03/02/health/02brod.html?module=Search&mabReward=relbias%3Aw&_r=1&), 1 March 2010.

4 'Younger Skin Through Exercise', *New York Times* (http://well.blogs.nytimes.com/2014/04/16/younger–skin–through–exercise/?module=Search&mabReward=relbias%3Aw), 16 April 2014.

5 P.T. Williams, 'Prospective study of incident age-related macular degeneration in relation to vigorous physical activity during a 7-year follow-up', *Investigative Ophthalmology & Visual Science*, January 2009, 50(1), pp.101–6.

6 'Even More Reasons to Get a Move On', *New York Times* (www.nytimes.com/2010/03/02/health/02brod.html?module=Search&mabReward=relbias%3Aw&_r=1&), 1 March 2010.

7 'Exercise: 7 benefits of regular physical activity', Mayo Clinic (www.mayoclinic.org/healthy–living/fitness/in–depth/exercise/art–20048389), accessed 28 October 2014.

8 '2008 Physical Activity Guidelines for Americans', Office of Disease Prevention and Health Promotion (www.health.gov/paguidelines), accessed 28 October 2014.

9 'The Scientific 7–Minute Workout', *New York Times* (http://well.blogs.nytimes.com/2013/05/09/the–scientific–7–minute-workout), 9 May 2013.

10 Personal communication by Susan Duffy, OSHA research consultant, July 2014, Washington, DC.

11 Caroline O.C. Werle et al., 'Is it fun or exercise? The framing of physical activity biases subsequent snacking', *Marketing Letters Journal*, 15 May 2014.

12 'Inadequate Sleep Can Lead to Obesity in Teens', *Nature World News* (www.natureworldnews.com/articles/8666/20140822/inadequate–sleep–lead–obesity–teens.htm), 22 August 2014.

13 M.P. St-Onge et al., 'Short sleep duration increases energy intakes but does not change energy expenditure in normal-weight individuals', *American Journal of Clinical Nutrition*, 29 June 2011.

14 K. Spiegel et al., 'Sleep Duration and Levels of Hormones That Influence Hunger', *Annals of Internal Medicine*, 7 December 2004, 141, pp.846–50.

15 'Stanford study links obesity to hormonal changes from lack of sleep', Stanford Medicine News Center (http://med.stanford.

edu/news/all–news/2004/stanford–study–links–obesity–to–hormonal–changes–from–lack–of–sleep.html), 6 December 2004.

16 'Losing Weight with Sleep Apnea', National Sleep Foundation (http://sleepfoundation.org/ask–the–expert/losing–weight–sleep–apnea), accessed 28 October 2014.

17 'Sleep loss boosts appetite, may encourage weight gain', University of Chicago Medicine press release (www.uchospitals.edu/news/2004/20041206–sleep.html), 6 December 2014.

18 'Obesity and Overweight', Centers for Disease Control and Prevention (www.cdc.gov/nchs/fastats/obesity–overweight.htm), accessed 28 October 2014.

19 University of Chicago Medicine, op. cit.

20 E.V. Cauter et al., 'The Impact of Sleep Deprivation on Hormones and Metabolism', *Medscape Neurology*, 2005, 7(1).

21 S.R. Patel et al., 'Association between Reduced Sleep and Weight Gain in Women', *American Journal of Epidemiology*, August 2006, 164(10), pp.947–54.

22 F.P. Cappuccio et al., 'Sleep duration predicts cardiovascular outcomes: a systematic review and meta-analysis of prospective studies', *European Heart Journal*, 2011.

23 'Sleep Disorders', Anxiety and Depression Association of America (www.adaa.org/understanding–anxiety/related–illnesses/sleep–disorders), accessed 28 October 2014.

24 M.P. St-Onge, op. cit.

25 'Is your insomnia down to what you are eating?' *Daily Mirror* (www.mirror.co.uk/lifestyle/health/your–insomnia–down–what–you–1919884), 30 May 2013.

26 K.G. Baron et al., 'Exercise to improve sleep in insomnia: exploration of the bidirectional effects', *Journal of Clinical Sleep Medicine*, 15 August 2013, 9(8), pp.819–24.

6 Practise Mindfulness (Chill Out)

1 'The Effects of Stress on Your Body', *WebMD* (www.webmd.com/balance/stress–management/effects–of–stress–on–your–body), accessed 28 October 2014.

2 'Treating Hypertension "Naturally"', *WebMD* (www.webmd.com/hypertension–high–blood–pressure/features/treating–hypertension–naturally), accessed 28 October 2014.

3 R.D. Brook et al., 'Beyond Medications and Diet: Alternative Approaches to Lowering Blood Pressure', *Hypertension* journal (http://hyper.ahajournals.org/content/early/2013/04/22/HYP.0b013e318293645f.full.pdf), 22 April 2013.

4 E. Ophir et al., 'Cognitive control in media multitaskers', *Proceedings of the National Academy of Sciences of the United States of America*, 15 September 2009, 106(37), pp.15,583–7.

7 Respect Yourself (Stop Beating Yourself Up)

1 P. Ekman and R.J. Davidson, 'Voluntary Smiling Changes Regional Brain Activity', *Psychological Science*, September 1993, 4(5), pp.342–5.

2 'Big Smiles, Longer Lives?', *Health* (http://news.health.com/2010/03/26/big–smiles–longer–lives), 26 March 2010.

About the Author

Joe Cross is a film-maker, entrepreneur, author and wellness advocate. He directed, produced and was the subject of the award-winning documentary *Fat, Sick & Nearly Dead*, which has been seen by more than 20 million people around the world. His first book, *The Reboot with Joe Juice Diet*, was a *New York Times* bestseller and has been released globally in multiple languages. It is credited with having accelerated the plant-based eating movement by media outlets, including the *Wall Street Journal*, *The Times* of London and *The Dr Oz Show*. His website, www.rebootwithjoe.com, has become an integral meeting place for a community of more than 1.5 million Rebooters worldwide. His second documentary film, *Fat, Sick & Nearly Dead 2*, focuses on how to stay healthy in an unhealthy world.

Index

OSHA exercise guidelines 130–1
overweight problem xi
PAG (Physical Activity Guidelines for Americans) 126
portion sizes 86
schools and community 110
sleep loss in adults 134–5
Standard American Diet (SAD) 60
sugar consumption xii
urticaria (auto-immune disease) 3, 5, 6, 18, 29, 31

vegan spicy parsnip celeriac soup 201–2
vegans 71
    vegan diet 69
vegetables
    benefits of 63
    rainbow approach to 25, 64
    and sleep 138
    spicy veggie scramble 199
    vegetable omelette 197
    washing 188
vegetarians 71
    and unhealthy choices 72
    vegetarian diet 69
volunteering 110–11, 117

wake-up red juice 191
walking
    as exercise 126, 127, 128, 129, 131
    and mindfulness 149, 151–2
    and self-nourishment 167
walnuts
    classic greens with lemon chicken 206–7
    vegan salad 203

Wansink, Professor Brian 42–3
    Mindless Eating 48, 84–5, 87, 96
    Slim by Design 232–3
websites 233
    Reboot community 10–11, 104–5, 143
weight gain
    fluctuations 6, 7–8, 11, 12, 13
    and food habits 85–6
    and self-respect 165–6
    and sleep loss 135
weight loss
    and community 113, 118, 119
    fluctuations 6, 7–8, 11, 12, 13
    Joe xv, 3, 4, 5, 8, 13
    Phil Staples 6, 30
    self-help groups for 107
    and sleep 132–3
    sustaining 16–17
weight regain 16
    Phil Staples 30, 33
weight training 126, 127, 128
willpower 20
women
    comfort food 43
    sleep loss and weight gain 135
worry journals 141

yoga 151, 157, 227
    planner 228–9
young adults
    sleep loss 134–5

zucchini
    courgette 'pasta' primavera 210–11

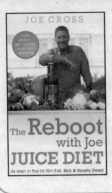
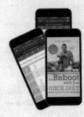
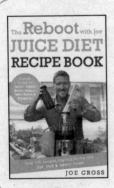